maps of the mind

How
Brains
Make Up Their
Minds

Maps of the Mind is a series of books by leading brain researchers from around the world, covering the major themes and topics in the sciences of the brain and mind. It is under the general editorship of Steven Rose, Professor of Biology at The Open University, UK.

The first four titles in MAPS OF THE MIND are:

Pain: The Science of Suffering
Patrick Wall

The Making of Intelligence
Ken Richardson

How Brains Make up Their Minds
Walter J. Freeman

Sexing the Brain
Lesley Rogers

Future contributors to the series include:

Enrico Alleva
Igor Aleksander
Ciaran Regan
Tim Halliday
Rusiko Bourtchouladze
James L. McGaugh
Lawrence Whalley

How
Brains
Make Up Their
Minds

Walter J. Freeman

Weidenfeld & Nicolson

LONDON

First published in Great Britain in 1999
by Weidenfeld & Nicolson

© 1999 Walter J. Freeman

A CIP catalogue record for this book
is available from the British Library.

ISBN 0 297 84257 9

Typeset by Selwood Systems, Midsomer Norton
Printed in Great Britain by Butler & Tanner Ltd,
Frome and London

Weidenfeld & Nicolson
The Orion Publishing Group Ltd
Orion House
5 Upper Saint Martin's Lane
London, WC2H 9EA

Contents

Acknowledgements

This book is based on my experimental data on brain function amassed over the course of half a century. Analysis of the data called for explanatory concepts drawn from neuroscience, psychiatry and neurology, and from other fields including physics, mathematics, statistics, psychology and philosophy, particularly the works of those who thought deeply about the nature of mind and behaviour. My problem was to translate some basic concepts in each of these fields into the others in order to bridge the gap between them, because any idea that can withstand serial translation between languages becomes clarified and strengthened. I have enjoyed conversations and debates with colleagues and students in many fields, and the creative criticism and editing of several assistants. Among many others I express my gratitude and appreciation to Hubert Dreyfus, Hermann Haken, Ilya Prigogine, Gianfranco Basti, Chris Cordova, Sean Kelly, Lillian Greeley, Paige Arthur, Leif Brown, Ken Thomas, Jennifer Hosek, Greg Keaton, John Barrie, Leslie Kay and Helen Cademartori, and to Chris Gralapp for illustrations. I have minimized citations to the literature to preserve the flow of thought. Full references are published in my earlier books in 1975 and 1995. I am pleased to acknowledge research support for four decades from the National Institute of Mental Health, and for the past decade from the Office of Naval Research. I dedicate the book to the memory of Hank Lesse and Dan Sheer. They gave their lives to '40 Hz', but nobody listened.

Chapter 1

Self-control and intentionality

Who is really in charge: you or your brain? And if it isn't your brain, who or what are you that you should have this power? The philosopher René Descartes conceived of the body, which includes the brain, as a machine piloted by the soul. According to this view, whether you call yourself a soul, a spirit, a free agent, or something else, you control your brain; or at least, you could or should if you have the knowledge and strength.

But recent developments in the brain sciences have called into question whether you or your brain actually have any control at all. Neurogeneticists claim that your genes determine not only the shape and colour of your body, but also your level of intelligence, your moods, your modes of sexual expression, and the frequency with which you use violence to achieve the goals assigned to you by your forebears, who blindly passed on their own genetic make-up. Neuropharmacologists see brains as chemical machines run by neuromodulators (hormone-like chemicals in brains that modify and fine-tune brain cells, the neurons). Having a mood disorder and turning to a neuro-psychiatrist for help is like having a broken-down car and not knowing how it works, and getting repairs from an expert whom you don't fully trust. At least these clinicians offer a scrap of liberty by admitting that you can choose whether or not to take their prescribed medicines. Even that small dignity is taken away by sociobiologists, who claim that if you take the pill, you are following the path of docility laid down for you in your early education, but if you refuse it, you are taking the fixed reflex path of rebellion against a tyrannical parent.

These doctrines of genetic and environmental determinism lie at the heart of the nature–nurture debate, that long-standing dispute over whether you behave the way you do because you were born that way or because you were raised that way. The problem with this argument is that it excludes the possibility that you can make your own contributions. It assumes that all your decisions are forced on you by your given circumstances. This deterministic reasoning is reminiscent of the theological doctrines of the predestinarians, who believed that their eventual disposition to heaven or hell had already been determined when the world began, so they were free to commit any sin and adopt any vice without affecting their personal outcomes. But they created their own hell on earth when their neighbours, objecting to such licentious and fatalistic behaviours as perversions of religious doctrine, invaded their communities to destroy them.

The fact is that we do make choices, even if it is only to avoid the opportunities to do so or to explain them away. We are not merely buffeted by circumstances like stones rolling downhill, as the philosopher Benedict Spinoza claimed in the seventeenth century. Every choice we make is deeply personal, arising in the entire past experience within each of us, not as a static collection of memories, but as a fabric of interlocked influences, desires, detestations and talents that constitute the meaning of everything we do. We all try constantly to clarify this flux and emphasize features that give the appearance of order and intelligibility to our turbulence, and we identify salient aspects as causes, determinants and rationales. We use reason to search for what we believe are the meanings of the objects, events and actions in our lives. It is very important to us that we explain our perceptions and actions in this way, so we can learn what to change in ourselves, our behaviours, and the world around us, and attain our personal goals more effectively.

Choices are chains of branch points by which each of our lives progresses, whether to a flowering realization of possibilities, or to a dreary dead end in a jail, a failed marriage, or a suffocating job. Looking back, if we succeed, we can praise ourselves, and if we do not, we can blame others. In looking forward to every choice, we try to understand what it is within ourselves or our brains by which we make decisions, either to go along an easy route or to defy predictions and shake off the dead hand of the past.

What is at issue is the nature of self determination. The problem boils down to the questions of how and in what sense brains, with their cells, the neurons, can create actions and thoughts, which we experience as our minds and ourselves, and whether or how our experiences can change or influence our brains and their neurons. What does it mean to say that one causes the other?

Many neuroscientists avoid these questions altogether. Those who are committed to full-blown nature–nurture determinism claim that our experience of self control in making choices is an illusion, and that our awareness of the process is a useless side effect, like the noise an engine makes while running, which these deterministic philosophers call an 'epiphenomenon'. They point to the impossibility of explaining in their materialistic terms how feelings and thoughts can break into the chains of chemical and electrical cause and effect that shape the activity patterns of neurons and the resulting patterns of muscular actions that we observe as behaviour. They say that such intrusions of mental events into the physical world, if they occurred, would be like miracles in the Middle Ages, acts in which God suspended natural laws for divine purposes. They regard psychological experiences of objects and events, which make up the contents of the stream of consciousness, as side effects.

Experiences of the redness of a sunset, the fragrance of a flower, or the song of a bird, which philosophers call 'qualia', are private and in their view are not accessible to scientists or worthy of scientific study. They claim that every form of behaviour is caused by a neural event in a brain, and that every such neural event has its prior cause in a combination of previous inputs to that brain. Their aim is to discover the natural laws by which stimuli are transformed and transported from the world by sensory neurons into brains and then processed to give predictable behaviours. In their view, there is room for chance, but not for choice.

A variant of this approach is to tinker with the idea of causality. Aristotle did this by defining four kinds of cause. For example, a statue has a material cause, which is the stone; a formal cause, which is its shape; an efficient cause, who is the sculptor; and a final cause, for the sake of which the work was done. This doctrine works well for man-made machines and works of art, but doesn't make sense when it is applied to the engineer or the artist. Brain matter is the chemical material of which it is made, and its form is the topic of neuroanatomy. The efficient cause of a brain is in its genes and its environment, and its final cause is biological destiny. The four-way breakdown leaves no room for the possibility of individuals and groups creating – causing – new ideas, devices and art forms. Aristotle left no room for the imagination.

Other brain scientists avoid the problem of how brains cause thinking by proposing that neural and mental events are different aspects of the same thing. This is known as the psychoneural identity hypothesis. It is like looking at a rabbit through the two ends of its tunnel. It may seem like a reasonable idea that is hard to dispute in principle because, after all, you can't think without having a functioning brain, and part of brain function is thinking, but there is no way to test it directly. On the one hand, whatever you may be thinking now, you cannot simultaneously go into your brain and observe your own brain activity while you are thinking it. On the other hand, no one else who is observing your brain activity can know exactly what you are thinking, even when you try to put your thoughts into words. Current studies in brain imaging show that different parts of brains are more or less active in various kinds of cognitive tasks, but the colour patches on the brain maps can't show what the thoughts are, so we have to accept the identity as an untestable theory. One person cannot see the head and tail of the rabbit in its tunnel at the same time, but two people can, and can agree that both exist, and that the views are not identical but the animal is. They can combine their visions using a theory about the rabbit to assemble a whole picture. But then causality isn't relevant, because the head and tail don't cause each other. According to rabbit theory, we think of them simply as parts of a whole.

Still, causality should not be omitted from brain theory. Some brain scientists, myself among them, are committed to a different point of view, in which the power to choose is an essential and unalienable property of human life. Instead of postulating a universal law of causality and then having to deny the possibility of choice, we start with the premise that freedom of choice exists, and then we seek to explain causality as a property of brains. This premise is not based in ethics. On the contrary, many ethical questions follow from this premise, such as whether freedom of choice is a good thing, in what circumstances it should be encouraged or refused, and who has the right to exercise it or to infringe it for others on the basis of gender, race, age, education and possession of property. We recognize that many, if not most, people in history have endured restrictions on exercising this right under social regimes that have been imposed upon them, and also that some of them have welcomed release from the accompanying responsibility. This premise has been the bedrock of Anglo-American democracy since the eighteenth century. But discoveries in biology and physics dating from the seventeenth century have for the most part been interpreted as denying this personal liberty. Spinoza claimed that the only difference between a man and a stone going downhill was that the man had the illusion that he had chosen to do so.

In this book, I hope to turn the biology around so that a proper understanding of brain dynamics supports and explains the biological capacity to choose. In order to do this, I have to meet three conditions. One condition is that we comprehend the brain mechanisms through which neurons construct the options from which we choose. Another condition is that we must explain what is happening in the organization of neurons in our brains at moments of choice. And the third condition is that we must explain in neural terms the nature and role of awareness and how states of awareness are linked in the sequence that provides the contents of consciousness. In other words, a foundation must be laid to understand and take charge of the functions of brains, in terms that are readily compatible with the facts of neuroscience and with the intuitions, thoughts and qualia by which we live our daily lives and make choices.

Even ten years ago, an attempt to lay such a foundation was impossible. Since then, though, we have seen the emergence and flowering of two new scientific fields. One of these new fields is brain imaging, by which the activity patterns of fields of neurons can be observed and measured during the course of normal behaviour. The images of the whole brain are dominated by activity patterns in the cerebrum, also known as the forebrain, and its outer shell, the cerebral cortex (Figure 1), but contributions also come from massive collections of neurons buried deep in each hemisphere, the basal ganglia, and from the brainstem, which connects the cerebrum to the cerebellum and spinal cord. The other new field is nonlinear brain dynamics, including those areas dealing with self organization in complex systems that are being studied by physicists, chemists and biologists, and with the endlessly new activity patterns to which they give rise. We now recognize these patterns as manifestations of chaos, which looks like noise but has hidden order and the capacity for rapid and widespread changes, just as our thoughts do. Noise, like the heat in an electric stove, is slow to start and stop. Chaos is like the movement of bodies in an airport terminal: patterns change at moments of announcements. Never before nonlinear dynamics have we been able to make the distinction between noise and chaos.

Both of these new fields have been made possible by the conceptual development and widespread availability of digital computers. The large body of literature on these topics is matched in magnitude by the enormous amount of information and literature about brains. I have simplified my task of describing a foundation for the analysis of behaviour in terms of chaos by limiting my analysis to just those aspects of theory and experimental findings on brain functions that bear on the prob-

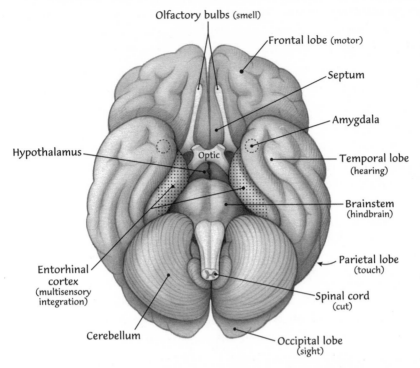

Olfactory bulbs (smell)

Frontal lobe (motor)

Septum

Amygdala

Hypothalamus

Optic

Temporal lobe
(hearing)

Brainstem
(hindbrain)

Parietal lobe
(touch)

Entorhinal
cortex
(multisensory
integration)

Spinal cord
(cut)

Cerebellum

Occipital lobe
(sight)

Figure 1 The brain as it appears from underneath. The two hemispheres of the cerebrum (the forebrain) have five lobes, of which only the frontal and temporal lobes and small parts of the occipital lobes are visible from below. The hemispheres are joined through the midbrain (not seen) to the brainstem and cerebellum. The medial temporal lobe, indicated by the stippling, contains the entorhinal cortex, which is the main source of input to the hippocampus located above it. These are major parts of the limbic system. Olfactory input goes directly into the entorhinal cortex from the olfactory bulbs, whereas all other senses go by roundabout stages through the brainstem to the basal ganglia and cortex, which is the outer shell of each hemisphere. The basal ganglia, which include the thalamus, are masses of neurons inside the forebrain that can only be seen by dissection.

lems of how brains make choices, and that determine when, how, and with what importance the 'I' of awareness is involved in the process.

I hope to encourage the belief that people have the power to make choices. I will do this by explaining the neural mechanisms through which goals emerge within brains and find expression in goal-directed actions. In my view, these mechanisms give rise to the conception of causality as a trait peculiar to humans.

There is no need to justify the concepts of either free will or universal determinism, because they and their irresolvable antinomy now seem to be the logical consequences of mistaken beliefs about causality.

If I can make clear how readily the new findings from neuroscience serve to strengthen ideas concerning self determination and individual responsibility, and if I can create a better understanding of how people choose to form social bonds, and why they do it in the ways they commonly do, then I will have achieved the aim of this book. To protect a free society from impediments imposed by resorting to the conceptual restraints of genetic and environmental determinism, we need to understand how our brains and bodies, given what they have to work with, shape themselves and make up who we really are, not merely who we think we are.

I will begin by giving a name to the process by which goal-directed actions are generated in the brains of humans and other animals. Such goal-directed actions would often be called 'voluntary' when they are done by humans but not by animals, because many people think that only humans have the capacity to will their actions. As an alternative to this understanding of volition, I want to describe a neural basis for goal-directed actions that is common to both humans and other animals, because it reflects the evolution of human mechanisms from simpler animals, in which intent can operate without will. The concept – 'intentionality' – was first described by Thomas Aquinas in 1272 to denote the process by which humans and other animals act in accordance with their own growth and maturation. An 'intent' is the directing of an action towards some future goal that is defined and chosen by the actor. It differs from a 'motive', which is the reason and explanation of the action, and from a 'desire', which is the awareness and experience stemming from the intent. A man shoots another with the intent to kill, which is separate from why he does it and with what feeling.

Lawyers following in the steps of Aquinas understand and use these distinctions. Psychologists commonly do not. Philosophers have drastically changed the meaning of the term, using intention to denote the relation that a thought or a belief has to whatever it signifies in the world, but physicians and surgeons, again following Aquinas, have preserved the original sense in applying the word to the processes of growth and healing of the body from injuries, thus retaining its original biological context. I believe that animals have awareness, but not awareness of themselves, which is well developed only in humans. Self awareness is required for volition: animals cannot volunteer.

In Chapter 2 I describe my conception of meaning, how it is created by the processes of intentionality, and how it is expressed in symbols, gestures and words comprising representations. I propose that meanings arise as a brain creates intentional behaviours and then changes itself in accordance with the sensory consequences of those behaviours. Aquinas and Jean Piaget both called this process 'assimilation'. It is the process by which the self comes to understand the world by adapting itself to the world. The contents of meaning derive from the impact of the world, principally the social impact of actions of other humans upon ourselves, and they include the entire context of history and experience we have already acquired. Although the contents of meaning are largely social in origin, the mechanisms of meaning are biological and have to be understood in terms of brain dynamics.

Meaning is a kind of living structure that grows and changes, yet endures. In Chapter 3 we shall address the problem of the origin of such structure through nonlinear dynamics. Structure comes from chaos, which is an expression of self determination. Here we need to grasp the hierarchical nature of the way neurons are organized at two levels of size and scale, including the concepts of the state of a neuron and of a neuron population in a brain, its state variables and state space, the stability of states, and state transitions between states through destabilization.

In Chapter 4 these concepts of dynamics will be applied to the first steps of perception following environmental impact onto the senses, in which the brain responds to the world by destabilizing the primary sensory cortices of the brain. The result is the construction of neural activity patterns, which provide the elements of which meaning is made. When the freshly made patterns are transmitted to other parts of the brain, the raw sense data that triggered them are washed away. What remains is what has been made within the brain. This process resembles digestion, in which food is broken down into molecules that are immunologically acceptable, and the parts are reassembled into macromolecules that have the unique imprint of the individual immune system. The dynamics isolates the meaning in each brain from all others, endowing each person with ultimate privacy, and loneliness as well, which creates the challenge of creating companionship with others through communication. I call this condition 'epistemological solipsism', to conform with the philosophical term for a school of thought that holds that all knowledge and experience is constructed by and within individuals. (This view differs from the extreme and discredited view called 'metaphysical solipsism', which holds that the whole world is a fantasy of each individual.) One aim in this book is to explain why this isolation must exist, and to discuss the mechanisms of constructing meaning and of inducing the construction of similar meaning in others, in order to overcome this isolation. How else can parents and children come to a satisfactory understanding after the years of teenage maturation and rebellion?

In Chapter 5, we shall see how the sensory portals cooperate with deeper structures in the brain to construct brain activity patterns in which inputs from all the senses are blended. This blending is the original meaning of common sense, rather than the street-smart worldliness that is often taken for folk wisdom. No one neuron or part of the brain takes charge to control the other parts. Coordination is invitational, not domineering. The key to brain function lies in the massive recurrent pathways by which each part of the brain broadcasts its output to other parts and receives from them, rather like singers in a chorus hearing and reacting to all the others. These interactions provide the basis for the neural consensus that is necessary for the self organization of behaviour.

In Chapter 6, we will look at the relation of awareness to

the formation and representation of meaning. Most intentional behaviours occur without the need for awareness, so intentionality operates before awareness and consciousness, up to a point. That point is reached when, in order to understand intentionality, we need to think about meaning and to represent our thoughts in words. We need to hear and read the words of others to enhance our own meanings. Effective use of language requires consciousness. We will approach the biology of consciousness by looking at the concepts of linear and circular causality. The way we think about causes can be explained in neurobiological terms as coming from the way we are aware of and experience our own intentionality. This step shows the limits of linear causality and helps us to understand circular causality, which is a kind of half-way house between the comfortable shelter of belief in causality and the rather terrifyingly inhuman open range of acausal processes. My conclusion comes to rest on a premise proposed by the psychologist William James in 1879, that consciousness is interactive with brain processes, and is neither epiphenomenal nor identical with those processes. Consciousness does not control behavioural actions, at least not directly. In terms of dynamics it is an operator, because it modulates the brain dynamics from which past actions sprang. Residing nowhere and everywhere, it reworks the contents that are provided by the parts. In humans, the exuberant growth of the frontal and temporal lobes (Figure 1) provides the mechanisms of self consciousness. Animals do not have these parts in their brains, and their behaviours give no evidence of self consciousness or self awareness. The possibility exists of being conscious without being self conscious or even being aware of intentional action.

In Chapter 7, we shall see how brains surmount solipsistic isolation and form societies, through which some contents of meaning are partially assimilated by the members of society and represented in knowledge. The most common method of assimilation of meanings is in the give and take of conversation. The deep formation of trust requires more complex behaviours, which involve the induction of altered states of consciousness, including trances. Among the many techniques used are behavioural aids such as chanting, drumming and dancing, with chemical aids such as alcohol and hallucinogens. The essence of these procedures is to loosen the self-conscious control of individuals and dissolve their cognitive and emotional structures in a meltdown of meanings that are counter to socialization. I call this process 'unlearning'. It is an essential precursor to new learning leading to socialization that takes place through cooperative and nurturing behaviours. Hints of the brain chemistry involved are found in the mammalian evolution of parental bonding to offspring that need prolonged care by adults in order to survive. Unlearning is mediated by neuromodulators in the brainstem, particularly oxytocin and vasopressin, which are released in brains during reproductive behaviours that include sexual intercourse, giving birth and nursing. My final conclusion is that consciousness, as it is understood among people for whom it is self evident, is a social contract that governs the ethical behaviours and attitudes we adopt with respect to people and all living things. Whatever it is in humans that makes the choices, it cannot fail to be a social being immersed in a cultural milieu from years of personal socialization and millennia of cultural history.

The questions raised in this book have been debated and answered provisionally for three thousand years according to the historical record, and probably for thousands of years before the development of writing. What allows us a fresh start now is our ability to image brain activity during normal behaviour, and to model our findings with the tools of nonlinear dynamics. However, these new data are being acquired under preconceptions embodied in old experimental designs, and we have to reinterpret them as they bring new concepts to light. It is hard for nonspecialists to grasp the elementary properties of neural activity, but it is even harder for specialists to unlearn old points of view to make way for new ones. One aim of this book is to show just how difficult such intentional state transitions can be, and why they are so challenging.

Chapter 2

Meaning, representation and intentionality

A fundamental and enduring human activity is the search for meaning. What we are looking for is not something we can define, because the form that meaning takes is unique for each person. Nor is it necessary to try to define it, because it is universally experienced in the joy of realizing it and in the pain of losing or lacking it. People seek meaningful relationships, experiences and causes. What distinguishes these from meaningless situations, chance encounters, and lost causes is a richness of context and the promise of a continuing emergence through our personal choices of interesting and fruitful complications.

Consider the meaning of a raised eyebrow. On a camping trip, it may be a defensive gesture against an annoying insect. At a dinner party, it may express surprise at the arrival of an unexpected guest, and joy if desired or dismay if unwanted. Between sexual predators it means something else, but what? He reaches with his hand to touch her elbow. She arches an eyebrow. Is this an invitation or an expression of contempt? He has to interpret the rotation of her body and the attitude of her head. She has to gauge his physical strength and pliancy of will. Their exchange of subtle signals has a purpose but is not deliberative, but automatic and habitual, a form of social negotiation of partly joint and partly conflicting aims and desires. Power? Companionship? Sex? Those aims invoke meanings in each of the pair, but the meanings are not the same. The meaning in each participant invests an entire personal history in the sequence of words and gestures between them.

Meanings have no edges or compartments. They are not solely rational or emotional, but a mixture. They are not thoughts or beliefs, but the fabric of both. Each meaning has a focus at some point in the dynamic structure of an entire life. Meaning is closed from the outside by virtue of its very uniqueness and complexity. In this sense, it resembles the immunological incompatibility of tissues, by which each of us differs from all others. The barrier between us is not like a moat around a castle or a fire wall protecting a computer system; the meaning in each of us is a quiet universe that can be probed but not occupied.

Brain scientists have paid little attention to how meaning comes into being, and what the conditions are that foster it. Some people passively expect it to happen to them, like the starving tramps in Samuel Beckett's play *Waiting for Godot*, who wait in the wilderness for one who never comes. For pragmatists and existentialists, it is clear that meaning forms through action. More specifically, it is created in and by their brains. My position is that we do not discover meaning in the way that we find exotic animals and minerals, through their serendipitous impact on our senses, nor do we invest it in the way we make deposits in bank accounts. Meaning is created in unique forms within ourselves through the actions and choices we all make, initially by learning to live according to a system of beliefs offered to us through our parents, peers or colleagues, first changed to suit ourselves, then modified to become ourselves. Every choice we make in everyday life is a way of grasping our part of the world we all cohabit, but in our own terms, in accord with our unique experiences.

Much of the effort and energy of our lifetimes is spent in trying to understand the meanings of others, and to induce others to understand our own. We can't ever fully transport or inject our meaning into anyone else, but we can express ourselves and invite communal actions as a way of bringing into harmony with others some part of the meaning structure within ourselves. We commonly speak of 'shared meaning' as though it could be distributed within a group, like food and wine. My belief is that meanings can be made to be similar in people who work, dance, sing and pray together, and I call this portion of their meaning structures 'assimilated meaning'. That fraction of assimilated meaning that can be represented as public knowledge suffices to support cooperation, although the meanings it leads to are never identical among the participants. The assimilated meanings are the basis for all knowledge in cultural, social and political groups, beginning with families.

The ways we communicate meaning include speech, facial expressions and gestures, as actors do, and by writing and making pictures, as artists do. These material forms are representations of meaning, but books, equations, movies and paintings have no meaning in themselves. They are capable of eliciting the construction of meanings in recipients and observers, but these meanings inevitably differ in each viewer from those of the authors and artists. We believe they have close resemblance, but they are unique to each of us.

So how, and in what sense, are meanings assimilated? One way is by successive approximations in conversation. Person 'A' expresses a meaning by making a representation of it, A1 (Figure 2). The receiver, 'B', creates a meaning and represents it by a statement, B1, such as 'I see what you mean', to which 'A' responds by modifying the meaning, and replies with a related representation, A2: 'No, I meant something a little different.' By repetition, a small area of correspondence forms between the meaning textures of the participants, an overlap that is confirmed by cooperative actions such as drinking together, which is the meaning of 'symposium'. When we act together we 'assimilate', which goes beyond 'correspondence' or 'congruency'. Words are merely cognitive, and cannot lead to the sense of trust that comes with deep assimilation of meaning. Joint action is the real glue that holds societies together. It begins with socialization in infancy and extends throughout life as the midwife of meaning in each of us.

People commonly suppose that meaning exists in natural events, such as sunsets, spring flowers and courtship displays

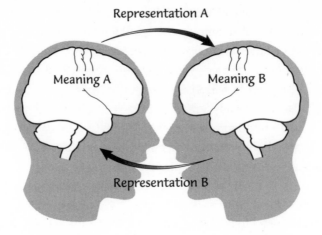

Figure 2 Meanings form in our brains. We make representations and use them to induce the formation of meanings in others. Most people think we attach meanings to representations (words, gestures, symbols and images) as carriers of meaning. Materialists and cognitivists also think that brains make representations inside themselves of the outside world and use these to store memories in the same way as computers, but they do not know how meanings are attached to their representations in either computers or brains. As a dynamicist and pragmatist, I propose that representations exist only in the world and have no meanings, and that meanings exist only in brains without being represented there.

by animals. In my view, the meanings exist in the observers, including the participant animals, and not in the objects, events and bodily motions. Brains alone have meanings, and they are very different from representations. In order to understand this difference, we need to distinguish between a mental representation and a mental state. During the past three hundred years, we have become accustomed to expressing our thoughts representationally. The metaphor 'mental image' has replaced the actual description of our experience of thinking, to the point that it may seem contentious to question the utility of the metaphor in understanding brain function. Yet the mental content that precedes the execution of a painting, a novel or a model, for example, differs profoundly from the forms that are frozen into the work. This is true of every act in comparison to its preceding mental state. When we seek to correlate a brain state with a behaviour, we should compare our measurement of a pattern of brain activity not with a mental concept in ourselves, but with a state of meaning that we infer exists in the brain of the person or other animal we are observing.

Because brains are composed of interconnected neurons, there must be some way in which meanings arise through the activities of neurons. We already know a great deal about the anatomy, physics and chemistry of neurons. What we most need now, to understand the relation of neurons to meaning, is a fresh perspective on the masses of data that neurobiologists have gathered, and on the puzzles those data pose. The old questions – How are voluntary actions generated? How does the firing of neurons give rise to awareness of meaning? How do brains make sense of the world? – remain challenging as neuroscientists test, observe and accumulate new data. But a new general theory to guide research in natural and artificial intelligence requires new assumptions and new definitions. I believe that the idea of meaning, a critical concept that defines the relation of each brain to the world, is central to current debates in philosophy and cognitive science, and will become so in neurobiology.

The process by which meanings grow and operate is intentionality. Most people understand 'intention' as referring to any conscious, goal-directed behaviour: 'I intend to eat lunch at noon'; 'I propose to go to the bank to get the money to pay for it'; 'The road to hell is paved with good intentions'. This everyday usage is a watered-down version of the concept devised by Thomas Aquinas. The other watered-down version has been used by philosophers in the past century to designate the relation between mental states and objects or events in the world, whether real or imaginary. A thought is always about something. A belief is always about some state of affairs. This use of intentionality is often referred to as the 'aboutness' of mental representations.

A major feature of both the everyday and recent philosophical usage of intentionality is an implicit requirement that mental states be conscious. However, we perform most daily activities that are clearly intentional and meaningful without being explicitly aware of them. Consider the activities of athletes and dancers, who move their bodies in space and time to some end (winning games, telling stories and expressing emotions). When people first learn to dance or play a sport, they draw upon conscious reflection of what they ought to be doing with their bodies, but mainly they draw unconsciously upon the already learned skills that we all have in using our bodies, such as running. As the training of the brain and body proceeds, that conscious reflection on the manipulation of the body falls away, and they can take the plunge through having what we commonly call a strong 'feel' for the game or dance. Performance becomes 'second nature'. For many people, the greatest fulfilment and enjoyment comes with total immersion into the activity, so that self awareness is scattered to the winds, and they become wholly what they desire in body and spirit, without reservation. The brain and body anticipate inputs, perceive, and make movements without need for reflection. It is precisely this kind of unconscious, but directed, skill in the exercise of perception that the concept of intentionality must include.

The examples of the athlete and dancer demonstrate what I consider to be the three main properties of intentionality. The first is unity. Our brains and bodies are entirely committed to the action of projecting ourselves corporeally into the world, and our perceptions are unified across all our senses at rates faster than we can perceive. Here I distinguish between the self, which is unified, and the awareness of self that we experience as the ego, which is not unified but can be splintered like sunlight on waves. The second property is wholeness: the entirety of life's experience is brought to each moment of action. The experiences of games and dancing are generalized and continually built upon. It includes an effort, described by Aristotle and again by Goethe two centuries ago, as a blind, organic striving towards realizing our full potential within the constraints of heredity and environment. The third property of intentionality is purpose or intent, because whether athletes and dancers are aware of it or not, their actions are directed to some end.

So perception is a continuous and mostly unconscious process that is sampled and marked intermittently by awareness, and what we remember are the samples, not the process. The fact that consciousness need not enter into the description of intentionality opens a new vista. Consciousness is not a good place to start a theory of brain function, because there is no biological test to prove whether consciousness is present in a supine subject, other than to ask 'Are you now or were you ever awake?'. Animals cannot answer, not because they can't remember or make representations in their own ways, but because they can't create and represent abstractions equal to the required level of sophistication of communication.

Evolutionary biologists have shown that complex operations of brains and bodies originate in simpler animals and have evolved into human capacities. Therefore, we can infer that animals have intentions by observing their behaviours, even if we do not know whether they are conscious of what they do. For example, an animal may wake up and, being hungry, go hunting. When it receives an odorant chemical representing food, it must extract and perceive an odour that it is searching for and distinguish it from the odorous background, which is an infinitely complex stew of chemicals that it cannot possibly identify and catalogue. Then it must search further to discover where the odorant is coming from. Conceiving the source is part of the meaning of the odour. To do this, the animal needs to know where it was when it perceived the odour, and needs to keep a record of how strong it was. It must determine the direction of the wind or water by the feeling on its skin, the sight of waving plants, and the sounds of the flow. On the basis of these new inputs, it must make another move, and it must know where it has arrived. It must get verification from the sensory receptors in its own muscles and joints of whether they have, indeed, done what the brain signalled them to do, or, if not, what they did instead. All of these inputs are combined into the unity of a multisensory perception, also known as a Gestalt, which provides the basis for what the animal chooses to do next. All these facets attach to the meaning of the perception, the odour, and none of them to the stimulus, the odorant.

The animal moves to a new location, takes another sniff and

compares the two odours. But the difference in strength between the two successive steps is meaningless unless the animal constructs a history of where it was on the first try and where it went on the second, by combining several multisensory perceptions that include its somatosensory records of body movements through its environment. This basic activity of the search for food demonstrates, once again, the three properties of intentionality. The hungry animal distinguishes its own body from external objects, such as potential food, and it keeps track of its movements in space and time, which shows a wholeness of experience. And its activity is tuned towards some end, a purpose, which is to satisfy its hunger, or to plan for the future by storing food, or to enjoy the food, or whatever. That is private, and we can only surmise what the animal intends from watching what it does.

I chose this example because everything that we know about our brains in comparison with those of other living animals and the fossil record tells us that biological intelligence evolved in the context of a brutal chemical arms race, the biological warfare of eat or be eaten. The nose was and is the first and final arbiter of what we ingest and of what we are afraid. Comparisons of brains show that the mechanisms of intentionality first emerged in the olfactory system, and that the visual, auditory and somatosensory systems moved in and co-opted the operating system, changing the details but taking advantage of the main thrust of the dynamics. Olfaction remains unique among the senses for the direct access its receptor neurons have to the cerebral cortex (Figure 1). This explains why odours of smoke, putrid flesh, coffee, tobacco, perfume, body odours and so on are so much more emotionally compelling than the visual and auditory sensations that accompany them. The lesson here is that we will not understand vision and hearing, including spoken and visual forms of representation, until we know how our brains cope with the infinite complexities of our olfactory environment.

The examples of the athlete, dancer and hungry animal return us to some fundamental questions. If the brain does not merely react to received stimuli, how do actions originate in the brain?

If the external world is infinite in the sensory stimuli that it gives to the body, how does the brain select what is of immediate importance for it? When awareness occurs, what is its biological nature, and what does it do? Is awareness necessary for meaning, and if so, in what way? Above all, how does the activity of neurons produce the unity, wholeness and intent that characterize intentional behaviour and meaning?

I wish to argue that these difficult questions have biological answers, and will begin by outlining my view of brain organization. There are two basic units: the neuron and the neuron population. The neuron is a specialized cell that acts upon another cell by transmitting an electrical pulse called an action potential, by which it releases a specialized chemical called a neurotransmitter. About 150 years ago, the medical sciences took a giant step forward when German physicians under Rudolph Virchow learned that all organs in the body are composed of cells. Modern medicine is built on what they called the 'cell doctrine'. It took another 50 years before neuroscientists became convinced that brains, too, are made of cells. For the past century, neurobiology has been based on the 'neuron doctrine' and the study of neurons one at a time.

However, just as important as neurons acting individually upon one another are masses of interacting neurons that form neuron populations, which have specific properties of their own that cannot be reduced to the level of the single neuron. Neuron populations have states and activity patterns just as neurons do, but they do different things. We call this population activity macroscopic to distinguish it from the microscopic activity of individual neurons. We will look at this in more detail in Chapter 3, but here we need to know about the existence of neuron populations. The world has effects on aggregates of microscopic neurons in sensory organs, which do not interact but individually send their action potentials into the brain. The brain acts into the world by microscopic motor neurons that send their action potentials to muscle cells. Between the non-interactive aggregates of sensory and motor neurons, it is the distinctive properties of neuron populations in our brains that enable us to deal with macroscopic things, like our bodies, the things we eat and build, and the people we love, attack or run away from.

Perception is organization of sensations and the construction of meanings, and this is what neuron populations do. When a microscopic receptor responds to a stimulus, such as an odorant, it transduces its input to an electrical current and then to action potentials that it sends to the brain, where macroscopic neuron populations create an activity pattern. This is, basically, the pattern of electrical brain waves recorded by an electro-encephalogram, or EEG. These macroscopic patterns, whatever they are, are crucial to understanding brain functions. My research has led me to believe that they are far more important than the conventional concept of neural function, the neuron doctrine, allows. Many researchers holding the conventional view think that neurons work like transistors in electronic net-works. That is an updated version of a century-old idea that a brain works like a telephone switchboard, according to which each sensory neuron transmits a signal that represents an object or a word in the environment, and the receiving neuron stores that signal for later use by switching its connections to other neurons. When a new stimulus arrives, a network of neurons compares it with the signals stored in the network to find the best match. The researchers call this pattern recognition, and think that population events, such as the EEG are irrelevant noise, like the sounds made by computers, which do not con-tribute anything significant. These neuron doctrinists have no concept of a macroscopic state.

This microscopic view fails to account for my data in at least two respects. First, a sensation from an odorant does not create a pattern in the brain that is fixed and stored away in a memory bank. Instead, I have observed that brain activity patterns are constantly dissolving, reforming and changing, particularly in relation to one another. When an animal learns to respond to a new odour, there is a shift in all other patterns, even if they are not directly involved with the learning. There are no fixed representations, as there are in computers; there are only mean-ings. Second, a sensory stimulus from an object does indeed induce the formation of a pattern in the brain, but when it is given repeatedly it does not induce precisely the same pattern in the same brain, let alone in any other brain. This is to be expected, because not only does the same object mean different things to different people, its meaning for the same person is continually shifting. My conclusion is that meaning cannot be transferred directly into and between brains in the way that information and knowledge based in representations can be transferred into and between machines. You can drill meaning into your children's brains about the piano keyboard and the multiplication table, but only if you induce them to practise, and then the forms are what the children make of them, not what you might want. You have to elicit meanings, and these are constructed and transmitted by the populations, not the individual neurons.

To relate the properties and operations of neurons and populations to the mental experience of meaning, I will contrast three modes of interpreting the experimental data we have from the neural and cognitive sciences about the nature of the mind. Within the general framework of the history of philosophy and psychology, there are three dominant views: materialist, cognitivist and pragmatist, of which my theory falls into the pragmatist category. We will look at these theories in order to get some useful vocabulary to interrelate neuroscience with philosophy and psychology.

The materialists view minds as physical flows, whether of matter, energy or information, which have their sources in the world. Minds are aspects of the flows happening in the brain that are causally linked, or even identical, to bodily processes. The materialist position traces its provenance to the Ancient Greeks, particularly to Hippocrates. Present-day materialists think of atoms and chemicals made of atoms, such as genes and enzymes, as the physical vehicles for the performance of brains and bodies, not materially different from plants and solar systems except in the way they are organized.

This approach has given us comprehensive bodies of data on the structure, chemistry and physiology of neurons and their development, and maps of their functional connections in sensory and motor systems. Materialists have repeatedly had striking successes in the past two centuries, notably in the use of chemicals to treat and prevent diseases from infection, malnutrition and aging, in the use of chemicals and surgical operations to modify and control behaviour, mood and emotional state, and in the proof that certain behavioural traits, such as mental deficiency or a tendency to depression, are under partial genetic control. Each of these successes demonstrates the potency of the materialist position.

As behaviourists and Pavlovian psychologists, they laid the basis for a materialist strain in holding that all behaviour is described by hierarchies of reflexes. Neurobiologists and physiological psychologists have changed the players in the materialist view to neural networks, computational assemblies, and hormonal pools of neurons, but they retain the stimulus–response determinism. For them, what is crucial is the activity of neurons, which are driven by stimuli, and which give neural commands for actions. Neurobiologists refer to these chains of cause and effect as information processing. They are started by stimuli that carry the information, and culminate in responses that convey transformed information. Simply put, brains process information by manipulating matter and energy.

The problem with this view is that it fails to account for the ways in which attention selects stimuli before they appear, or for the flexible specification of figures embedded in infinitely complex backgrounds – the face that leaps out at you in a crowd – or for the dependence of perception on action, or for the impact of our emotions on our qualia. Philosophers have played on these limitations by asking how the meaningless firing of neurons can give rise to meaningful experiences, such as pain, fear, rage and so forth, or even be identical with them. Although it is possible by brain imaging to describe the neural activity of a person in pain, and to find which parts of the brain can be stimulated to produce behaviours that manifest pain and various emotions, such descriptions do not answer a question that goes straight to the core of inner experience: 'What does it mean?'. Consciousness is not a problem for materialists, because they regard it as a functional state that can be suppressed, altered or restored by drugs. They address meaningful behaviours by the archaic, quasi-religious word 'voluntary', which is used in all modern textbooks on neurology and neuroscience to label actions that don't look like reflexes. That sweeps them under the epistemological rug, because the authors cannot explain how they arise.

The cognitivists argue that minds are made not of energy or matter, but of collections of representations that constitute symbols and images. They are software running on 'wetware'. Like materialism, this form of idealism also originated in Ancient Greece. Plato believed that a world of ideas existed apart from matter, which contained a fixed set of ideal patterns, a kind of supergeometry that guided the physical forms of matter that were realized as imperfect copies. It was up to the human intellect, through its power of reflection, to gain access to and comprehend the ideal forms by contemplating these shadows of reality. René Descartes elaborated this view by adding the notion of the primacy of thought in proving his own existence in the world. Then Immanuel Kant revolutionized Descartes' idealism by positing ideal forms of intuition that are innate to the mind, not to the world. According to Kant, all we are ever able to know about the world is filtered through our senses and organized by these innate categories. Processes that rely on the senses prevent us from knowing the world as it actually is. Therefore, we know the world only in terms of the representations synthesized in our minds. Categories are as close as we can get to the world as it really is.

Cognitivists have also been enormously successful in developing machines for information processing, and their view is quite popular today in various fields. Noam Chomsky's approach to linguistics is an excellent example. Chomsky believes that there are 'deep structures' laid down in brains, which provide an innate logical structure to all languages and which are implemented in differing details in various societies and cultures. Another example is artificial intelligence, or AI as it is often called. In the 1940s, neurobiologists and logicians reconceptualized the functions of neural activity. They conceived of neurons as binary switches performing Boolean algebra and forms of Aristotle's logic. Action potentials of neurons were no longer interpreted as electrical pulses, but as bits of information, binary digits that represented on or off, yes or no, one or zero. This led rapidly to the development of programmable digital computers, all starting from a mistaken view of how neurons work.

Information, according to the cognitivists, is carried by symbols that are manipulated according to prescribed rules. When they apply this doctrine to brains, they deduce that information is given by stimuli from the environment. It is encoded in trains of action potentials as bits that represent qualities, aspects or features of the stimuli. The features are transmitted by axons that serve as channels to the brain, where they undergo binding into representations of the stimuli by synaptic networks of neurons acting as summing junctions and logical gates. The contents are stored in memory banks as representational fixed patterns. They are recalled by being read out like the content-addressable memories in computers, so they can be matched or correlated with representations of new inputs. The important consequence of this conception is that information replaces energy and matter as the carrier of the flow of ideas. But information theorists have made it explicit that the information is divorced from meaning. What is crucial is not the content of a telephone call, but its bandwidth and the number and timing of the bits required to transmit the message. If this sounds a lot like the materialist view, that's because, over the past 50 years, neurobiologists have borrowed many of their interpretations of their data from cognitive scientists when they began to realize that the neuron doctrine wasn't working very well.

Cognitivists following this approach to construct artificial intelligence face a difficult problem, because they do not know how to attach meanings to the symbolic representations in their machines. The problem stems from their understanding of intentionality as 'aboutness', the relation to the world of the symbols that represent thoughts and beliefs about the world. Awareness is implicit in thinking and representing. Some biological systems have consciousness but, as Franz Brentano pointed out, so far, inanimate machines do not, because they do not have intentions. But what is the nature of consciousness? How is it made by brains? How might it be made to operate in artificial-intelligence brains to bring about changes in the machine parts and in the behaviour of the entire system? There is a great deal of debate within the cognitive-science community concerning precisely these issues. Consciousness is a great mystery. The problems are intractable because, in the field of cognitive science, meaning is defined by a relation between symbols, as in syntactical definitions of words by other words and pictures in dictionaries. But in reality, references to the world are not defined within a dictionary or a computer.

The third view of mind is pragmatism. Pragmatists think that minds are dynamic structures that result from actions into the world. In 1272, Aquinas introduced Aristotle to Western Europeans, particularly in his *Treatise on Man*, and to Aristotle's doctrine of active perception, according to which the organism learns about the world and realizes its potential by its actions on the world. Aquinas changed this concept to make it conform with Christian doctrine by distinguishing between will and intention. The will makes voluntary ethical choices in respect to good and evil, or right and wrong, and is something only humans have, whereas intention is the mechanism by which the potential of the organism is realized, something that other animals have, too. Aquinas further proposed that each animal is a unified being enclosed within a boundary that distinguishes 'self' from 'other', and that the self uses the body to push its boundary outwards into the world. Etymologically the word 'intend' comes from the Latin word *intendere*, which means not only to stretch forth, but equally importantly to change the self by experiencing action and learning from the consequences of acting.

Aquinas replaced Plato's idealism with Aristotle's materialism as the foundation of medieval church doctrine, but with a

brilliant distinction. For both Aristotle and Aquinas, but unlike
Plato, whom Aquinas severely criticizes, perception is an active
process, not the passive acceptance of forms. But for Aristotle,
the interaction of mind and world works in both directions.
Transitive actions, such as probing, cutting and burning, are
directed into the world as exploratory manipulations, and
stimuli thereafter enter into the body as the forms of material
objects. Intransitive actions are to understand and know the
forms of the objects through association. Aquinas concluded
from his conception of the unity of the self that the process is
unidirectional. Actions of the body exit by the motor systems,
changing the world and changing the relation of the self to the
world. The sensory consequences of the actions then enable the
body to change itself in accordance with the nature of the world.
However, the perception is only of the altered contours of the
self as experienced inside. No forms are pushed through or across
the boundary. The key word he used is 'assimilation' (*adaequatio*
means towards, but not at, equality). The body does not absorb
stimuli, but changes its own form to become similar to aspects
of stimuli that are relevant to the intent that emerged from
within the brain.

The process was likened by Aquinas to an observer shining a
light on the inside of a structure, such as a tent. The observer
infers what is happening outside from the patterns of reflected
light and the movements of the tent walls. But this is different
from the walls of Plato's cave, in that for Plato the light and
forms come from outside and are imperfectly caught by the
senses from the shadows on the passive wall, whereas for
Aquinas the forms are created inside the self through achieving
similitude. For example, when you shape one hand to hold a
coffee pot and adapt the other to hold a cup in order to fill it,
you do not transfer geometric shapes into your brain. Instead,
you incorporate your body to the forms of the objects by shaping
your hands to them, so you can manipulate them. The meanings
of the objects then grow in accordance with what you have done
with them and what you intend to do next, perhaps to taste,
drink or offer a cup to someone else. Other people can watch

what you do and learn by imitation, so their meanings are similar to yours but are homegrown, not transplanted.

Aquinas based his view of this unidirectionality on the incompatibility between the forms of matter, which are unique and particular, and the forms of intellect, which are generalizations and abstractions. These intellectual constructs are all that we can know, because each material object is infinitely complex in its details. No two cups are identical, even from the same mould. We merely imagine that they are for ordinary purposes. Forms are relative to scale. Razor blades all look like a straight line to the naked eye, but under an electron microscope each one looks like a different mountain range. Aquinas dissolved the dichotomy between subject and object, because the self creates its unique forms by its assimilation to the world, not by the discovery within itself of ideal forms, categories or eternal truths that are opposed to objects in the world. In contemporary terms, the body and the brain are open systems with through-put of matter, energy and information, but the unidirectionality of perception makes the fabric of meaning a closed system.

The world is infinitely beyond our limited powers of creating forms, and its particulars are inaccessible and useless for us. Are all hydrogen atoms identical? We cannot know, and do not care. The visionary poet William Blake wrote: 'If the doors of perception were cleansed, everything would appear to man as it is, infinite.' We know now that we would not perceive anything, because we would be overwhelmed. The process of intentionality, when it is working well, allows us to take in just as much as we can handle, and no more. When we are fatigued or mentally deranged, we suffer disintegration, what cognitivists call information overload. Our unidirectional perceptual system is our best asset in matching our limited capabilities to the infinite world.

Intentionality in the doctrine of Aquinas does not require consciousness, but it does require acting to create meaning instead of just thinking. This view is shared by the philosophers Martin Heidegger, Maurice Merleau-Ponty, J. J. Gibson, and the pragmatists. We sniff, move our eyes, cup an ear, and move our

fingers to manipulate an object in order to optimize our relation
to it for our immediate purpose. Merleau-Ponty called this
dynamic action the search for maximum grip, which is the
optimization of the relation of the self to the world by positioning
the sense receptors towards the object intended. His conception
is equivalent to Aquinas' assimilation. John Dewey described
the process as 'acting into the stimulus' and incorporating it into
future action, as distinct from merely reacting to it. Jean Piaget
based his analysis of psychological development on the concept
that infants learned very early about their bodies and their environments by active exploration, which he called 'the cycle of
action, assimilation, and adaptation' in what he identified as the
'sensorimotor' stage of early childhood, when infants constantly
move their bodies, especially their hands and feet, and drink
in the sensations they collect. Esther Thelen developed this
approach in the context of dynamic systems theory. Gibson
emphasized the 'affordances' of objects, by which he meant their
utility in respect to the purposes of the perceiver. He believed
that each object contained within itself the information that
showed how it was to be used. This information was extracted
by the brain through 'resonance' within brain systems, when
that information 'in-formed' the mind. His concept is also
equivalent to assimilation. He used these technical terms as
metaphors, because he had no neural mechanisms in mind, but
the terms convey the underlying idea of the unidirectionality of
perception in a finite being coping with an infinite universe.
That philosophical insight is crucial for interpreting my observations in experiments on neural mechanisms of perception in
animals.

Pragmatism has repeatedly failed to take centre stage in the
neural and cognitive sciences because it poses a major problem.
If minds are actions into the world, how are these actions generated? According to both the materialist and cognitivist views,
an action is ultimately determined by the form of a stimulus. A
laboratory rat can be trained to sit inertly until it is provoked. A
computer terminal waits for instructions from a user before
it acts. But wild animals and children don't wait. They are

continually engaging the environment, seeking stimuli with their own expectations and designs. Where in brains do endogenous actions of search and observing come from? How do brains generate them? Materialists and idealists for centuries, even for millennia, have appealed to myths of external powers that drive us, such as the Sun, moonbeams, the Big Bang, universal databanks, icons, totems, possessive demons, the world energy that Chinese physicians call *qi*, the orgone of Wilhelm Reich, and the connections to the spirit world by trees planted in sacred places, now transmogrified into nerve energy and the power of charismatic preachers. What do pragmatists have that can replace these compelling metaphors of energy driving us from outside? They have self organization, meaning that the self organizes itself. We drive ourselves? Yes, but how can neurodynamics measure up to the appeal of Cartesian soul?

Humans evolved from simpler creatures, and these earlier forms exhibit precursors of our rich and varied intentional behaviour. Evolution has given us the capacity to detect intentionality in others without needing to define it. We recognize directed behaviour almost instantly when we see it. When we encounter an object of a certain kind, we ask whether it is alive or dead, likely to attack or ready to escape if we try to capture it. If it is still, we ask if it is watching us. If it is moving, we ask if the motion is directed towards or away from us, or to other parts of its environment. In the modern world, we have little difficulty in distinguishing the behaviours of intelligent machines that do not know what they are doing from those of intentional animals that do. There are many examples in the zoological literature of intelligent behaviours exhibited by other vertebrates, and also invertebrates such as the octopus, bee or lobster. Charles Darwin found clear evidence for intentional behaviour in earthworms, and some scientists believe that even bacteria display it. My approach has been to study the brains of vertebrates that are simpler than humans, but not too simple or too different, because the appropriate simpler brains can start us on a well-marked trail in stages to human brains.

The brain of the tiger salamander, *Ambystoma tigrinum*, has been described by the comparative neurologist Charles Judson Herrick as being closer to that of our earliest vertebrate ancestor than any other existing brain. Its simple structure provides us with an introduction to brain function. I have adapted Herrick's view in Figure 3 to show the three main parts of the salamander brain: the forebrain, with its two hemispheres; midbrain; and the hindbrain, with its rudimentary cerebellum. The midbrain and hindbrain form the brainstem, which connects the forebrain to the spinal cord and the peripheral nervous system (not shown), which connects the sensory and motor nerves to the skeletal muscles, as well as the collections of neurons making up the autonomic nervous system, which regulates our vegetative functions.

In each hemisphere of the forebrain there are three main parts to the cortex. The anterior third takes care of sensory input. The most direct and dominant sense is that of smell, but some input comes from all the other senses (vision, hearing, taste and touch) by relays through the brainstem. The lateral part of each hemisphere (PC) is a motor cortex, which shapes bodily action. The medial part (H) is an association area, where inputs from all the senses are combined with one another into a field that provides for orientation in space and time.

Intentional action is directed by internally generated goals and takes place in the time and space of the world shared with other intentional beings. The materialist and cognitivist terms for these space–time processes are the short-term memory and the cognitive map. In the pragmatist view, these terms are misleading, because there is no temporary storage of images, and there is no representational map. One of the problems faced by pragmatists is to give biological content to the metaphors of memory, cognitive map, command and feature. These combined functions, however they are labelled and conceived, provide the tiger salamander with its space–time field of action, which is built into each of the intentional states it constructs. That field enables it to go to sites of expected reward, track a moving prey, or spot a hidden refuge. This association area in the salamander's brain is the forerunner of our hippocampus (Figure 1), which has

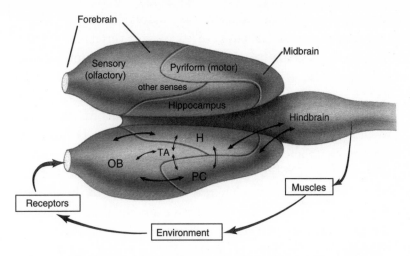

Figure 3 The forebrain is the organizing focus of intentionality in vertebrates. The simplest living example, in salamanders, has three essential components: sensory cortex, motor cortex, and association cortex (labelled here as the hippocampus, H). The basic architecture of these parts endures through the evolution of brains to mammals and humans as the limbic system. In most vertebrate brains, it is dominated by olfaction, but in human brains it is overgrown in much the same way that an ancient town is transformed by its modern suburbs without losing its core significance and street plan.

prominent roles in learning, spatial orientation, and remembering. Taken together, the sensory, motor and association cortices form a ring of interconnected neural tissue around a small central area, marked 'TA', which Herrick called a 'transitional zone'. He conceived this zone as the site of future growth and enlargement for the emergence of new parts in more advanced brains, particularly the mammalian neocortex. Yet these three primitive parts of the hemisphere have persisted as the limbic system (from the latin *limbus* meaning 'belt') around the stalk of each hemisphere connecting it to the midbrain. I will return to this topic in Chapter 5.

Researchers have studied the effects on behaviour of damage from disease or experimental surgery in many vertebrates, including salamanders, frogs, dogs and humans. The results show that the limbic system is essential for all intentional actions, including perception and most forms of learning. When a surgeon

cuts the connections between the brainstem and the hemispheres (Figure 1) and isolates the limbic system, an animal loses
all intentional behaviour. It retains the capabilities for chewing
and swallowing food put in its mouth, for locomotion with its
several types of gait, and for a variety of other regulatory functions called homeostasis by Walter Cannon, but it does not do
anything or go anywhere intentionally. The parts of the brain
that produce the patterns that orient activity into the environment are lost, and the capacities to execute the motor patterns
remain without direction. On the other hand, when the surgeon
removes any or all other parts of the forebrain deriving from
Herrick's transitional zone, the behaviour of the animal is
severely impoverished, because the animal is deaf, blind or partially paralysed, but its remaining behaviour is unmistakably
intentional.

The relations among the three parts of this simple brain are
crucial for understanding how they create intentional behaviour.
In each hemisphere, the sensory cortex receives input, the motor
cortex implements action, and the hippocampus provides multisensory integration and orientation in space and time. Each part
has reciprocal connections to the others (Figure 3). The entire
hemisphere constructs goal states through its interactive neural
activity patterns. Those patterned activities guide the body
through complex sequences of actions, and prime the sensory
cortex to select the smells, sights, sounds and tastes that are
predicted as the consequences of the impending goal-directed
actions. This is a central process that we call preafference, and
it provides the basis for what we experience as attention and
expectation. It enables the sensory cortices to predict specifically
how the actions to be taken will change the relations of the eyes,
nose, ears and fingers to the world. The messages are called
corollary discharges. Together they help us to distinguish
between changes in the environment and apparent changes that
are due to the intentional movement of our bodies, so that when
we move our eyes, we do not perceive the world to move. They
tell us whether the voice we hear, the hand we see or the odour
we smell is our own or someone else's.

The somatosensory cortex also receives messages from the muscles and joints, confirming whether an intended action has been performed, but this process of feedback is called proprioception, to distinguish it from exteroception of the world and interoception of the internal organs. Proprioception and interoception differ from preafference and corollary discharge by going from the brain through the body, instead of remaining entirely within the brain. For all cortices, preafference is the process by which we imagine what things may be like, if or when they come. The primary sensory cortices transmit their activity constantly and, if they have nothing to report, they transmit to our limbic system whatever their priming has led them to construct. The sensory receptors do not have that kind of selective autonomy for pattern formation. Cortices give visions and hallucinations. Receptors give itches and ringing in the ears.

The burning of fuel to maintain the metabolic ground state of your body and brain depletes your reserves and makes you hungry. As a hungry animal, you seek an odour of food by sniffing. When you locate it, you hold that smell, move your head and body, take another sample, and compare it with the first. Is it stronger or weaker? Do you go left, right or straight ahead? To decide that, you must know where you were, where you are now, what you did to get from there to here, and how long you took. Even this simple intentional task requires your brain to direct all sensory-induced activity patterns into the space–time field in the hippocampus to confirm or deny the expected consequences of each action, so each part of the brain is constantly interacting with the others. The assembled activity is unified, whole and purposive.

As animals evolve in competition for resources, their success depends on increasing the range and complexity of their possible courses of action and constructions of meaning. Brains increase in size and the complexity of connections. The dynamics of the activity comprising meanings require increasingly elaborate stages between the primary sensory cortices and the limbic system, while preserving the basic feedback interactions. In humans, these new stages may become well known because of their accessibility by non-invasive brain imaging: the cingulate, inferotemporal and orbitofrontal cortices. The new parts and connections provide ever greater sophistication, forming the basis for language, mainly in the left lateral hemisphere, and for social behaviour, through enormous expansion of the ventral frontal lobes. Singular destruction of these 'add-ons' can lead to blindness, deafness, partial paralysis, loss of language, and the 'social blindness' that is characteristic of damage in the frontal lobes. Yet intentional behaviour persists, albeit with impoverished meanings, unless there is also destruction in the limbic system, as in advanced Alzheimer's disease, which has a particularly virulent predilection for destroying the final link of the sensory cortices to the hippocampus. But singular destruction of the medial temporal lobes in both hemispheres does not abolish all aspects of intentionality. Instead, it results in loss of space–time orientation and the ability to add new episodic memories, that is, unity and wholeness. Goal-directedness is not restricted to the limbic system by any means.

These, then, are the issues I raise in this book: how patterns of brain activity are directed intentionally towards external objects, leading to the creation and assimilation of meaning through learning. The specific properties of neuron populations explain how the patterns arise and how they guide behaviour into the world by coordinating the firings of the microscopic motor neurons. I view the neural populations that compose the limbic system as the key to understanding the biology of intentionality. Paul Maclean called the limbic system 'the reptilian brain', implying that it is nasty and brutish with no respectable cognitive function. On the contrary, I think the limbic system is the principal director of action in space–time.

In the following chapters I will describe ten building blocks that allow us to understand how neural populations sustain the chaotic dynamics of intentionality, because the dynamics provides the biological basis for the flexibility, creativity and meaning of human behaviour. As a preview, the ten steps are listed here. Terms in bold are technical words that are required to name previously unknown objects and processes that have been disclosed by brain imaging and neurodynamics.

1. The **state transition** of an excitatory population from a point attractor with zero activity to a **non-zero point attractor** with steady-state activity by **positive feedback** (Figure 8).

2. The emergence of **oscillation** through **negative feedback** between excitatory and inhibitory neural populations (Figure 9).

3. The state transition from a point attractor to a **limit cycle attractor** that regulates steady-state oscillation of a **mixed excitatory–inhibitory cortical population** (Figure 10).

4. The genesis of **chaos** as **background activity** by combined negative and positive feedback among three or more mixed excitatory–inhibitory populations (Figure 11).

5. The distributed wave of chaotic dendritic activity that carries a spatial pattern of **amplitude modulation** made by the local heights of the wave (Figure 12).

6. The increase in **nonlinear feedback gain** that is driven by input to a mixed population, which results in construction of an amplitude-modulation pattern as the first step in perception (Figure 13).

7. The **embodiment of meaning** in amplitude-modulation patterns of neural activity, which are shaped by synaptic interactions that have been modified through learning (Figure 14).

8. **Attentuation** of microscopic sensory-driven activity and **enhancement** of macroscopic amplitude-modulation patterns by **divergent–convergent** cortical projections underlying solipsism (Figure 15).

9. The divergence of corollary discharges in **preafference** followed by **multisensory convergence** into the entorhinal cortex as the basis for Gestalt formation (Figure 17).

10. The formation of a sequence of **global amplitude-modulation patterns** of chaotic activity that integrates and directs the intentional state of an entire hemisphere (Figure 18).

These building blocks are heavy and difficult to grasp, but they are essential for understanding how brains make up their minds.

| # Dynamics of neurons and neuron populations

The brain, like all the other organs in the body, is an integrated assembly of cells, each of which is a semi-autonomous agent. In that respect, each cell is rather like a person in a society, being infinitely complex and unable to function, or even exist for long, except in the context of the whole. Rudolph Virchow's cell doctrine and its derivative, the neuron doctrine, are currently the bedrock for understanding neurons and the way they relate to one another. People who want to know how brains make minds need to concern themselves with the properties of the neurons that make up brains. In most respects, a neuron is a cell like any other cell: it is completely enclosed by a membrane, its genetic material is in a nucleus embedded in cytoplasm, and it is powered by its metabolic power packs, the mitochondria. Unlike other cells, however, the neuron sends out two kinds of threads that are extensions of its membrane. One kind is a dendrite, which looks like a bush or tree. A neuron typically has several main dendritic branches, each dividing repeatedly. The other kind of filament is an axon, one to a neuron, which also branches extensively. Input comes to the neuron through its dendrites, and output leaves the neuron through its axon. Both dendrites and axons grow extensively with no further cell division after birth (Figure 4), and axons in particular can stretch for remarkable distances, as though you could reach ten kilometres with one arm. These threads are the main difference between brains and other organs, such as the liver.

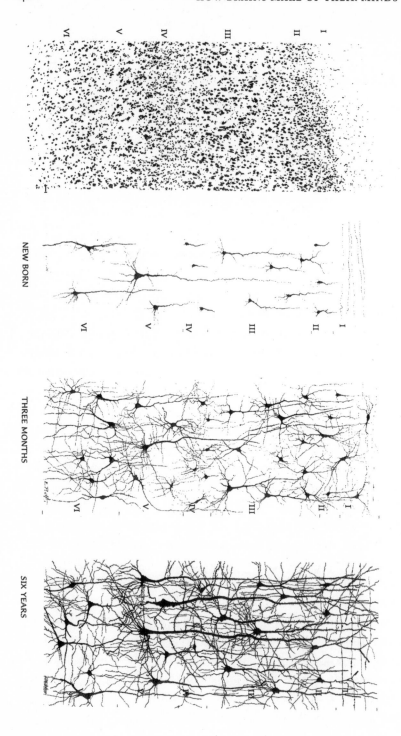

Figure 4 Neuropil is a tissue that consists of densely packed cell bodies (top) of neurons and filaments of their janitorial supporting cells called glia. The cells grow dendrites and axons like trees with intertwined branches that provide the large surface area of membrane needed to allow as many synapses as possible. New connections grow throughout life, mostly without adding more neurons. Synaptic connections are continually changed (formed, strengthened, weakened or deleted) through learning. The illustrations are from humans. In the top frame, each dot shows the nucleus of a neuron, like stars in a galaxy. The three lower frames reveal only 1 in 100 neurons to show the architecture of their branches. The neurons are too densely packed in neuropil to show more than this small fraction. The Roman numerals denote the conventional six layers of neurons in the neocortex which is a few millimetres thick; each cubic millimetre holds many thousands of neurons. Reprinted by permission of the publisher from *The Postnatal Development of the Cerebral Cortex* by J. L. Conel, Cambridge, MA; Harvard University Press. Copyright © 1939–1967 by the President and Fellows of Harvard College. Volume I, Plate L; Volume III, plate LVI; volume VIII, plates LXXXIV and LXXXVI.

There are two main types of neuron in the cerebral cortex. Projection neurons have a dendritic arbor that can grow to a diameter of up to a millimetre. Its main dendritic branch extends toward the surface of the cortex. There are also three or four basal trunks extending parallel to the surface, reaching out to adjacent neurons. The axon of a projection neuron extends beyond the dendritic arbor to other areas of cortex within each hemisphere, from one side of the brain to the other, and to targets in the brainstem and spinal cord. Remarkably, the axon can extend nearly half the length of a person's body, generally up to a metre in humans. Near where it leaves the cell body it has side branches, called axon collaterals, to other neurons nearby. The second type of neuron is the local neuron, or interneuron, whose dendrites form a densely branched arbor extending out in all directions to a diameter of about a tenth of a millimetre, or roughly 25 to 50 times the diameter of the cell body. These two types of neurons could be compared to road systems. The interneuron, in this analogy, is like the local streets, providing connections within a neighbourhood of neurons, whereas the projection neuron, like a system of main roads, provides the long-distance connections across the brain and to the spinal cord.

Neurons need extensive axonal branching if they are to send their pulses to as many other neurons as possible. Each neuron keeps the integrity of its membrane over all of its filaments, and its axon tips make contact with other neurons by forming bulbous enlargements that typically attach to the dendrites of other neurons at junctions called synapses. In the overwhelming majority of instances, the many synapses maintained by any one neuron on other neurons have the same effect on their targets, either increasing or decreasing the target activity, so in the following discussion we shall refer to them as excitatory neurons or inhibitory neurons to denote the effects they have. Most projection neurons in the forebrain are excitatory, whereas inter-neurons can be either excitatory or inhibitory.

There are several thousand synapses on the dendritic tree of each neuron. They take up space, which explains its tree-like structure, because the tree provides the surface area for as many contacts as possible, while giving every synapse a direct path to the axon near the cell body, by which the neuron gives output. The growth of dendritic trees continuously adds new surface area for more contacts, not only in childhood but also into adult life, even into healthy old age, as shown by Marian Diamond. Axons and their lateral branches also grow and divide, connecting with other neurons. The competition for synaptic space is intense, and success in finding and maintaining a connection depends on the synapses being active. If they are inactive, owing to damage or disuse, the connections decay and the synapses disappear. Even the neurons may vanish. The health of neural connections in old age, like muscles, requires exercise. The lifelong growth and the maintenance of active connections provide the basis for learning, remembering and adapting through modifications of the numbers and strengths of synapses, and they require daily exercise.

To describe the activities of neurons, we need a proper language, which is provided by the language of dynamics, the study of change. A neuron in its lifetime is active in a variety of states, such as rest, varying degrees of being excited or inhibited, and being changed by learning. The group of all possible states is called the state space of the neuron. The state space does not refer to an actual physical space, but rather to a range of possible states, rather like the psychological range of an individual who experiences varying degrees of alertness, fatigue, contentment and distress. A succession of states of a neuron form a pathway through its state space called a trajectory, such as from rest to excited to inhibited to rest again. Each neuron has certain pre-ferred trajectories that resemble habitual pathways, which Ichiro Tsuda calls its itinerancy, in an analogy to travelling salespeople going on their rounds. We can learn to predict such itinerant behaviour of neurons by observing them repeatedly. The neuron lingers for brief or extended time periods in each state throughout its itinerancy, always returning to its basal or resting state.

Given that the state of the neuron is subject to change, we describe the changes using state variables. Just as there are numerous parameters in human psychology, each aspect of the neuron that we can observe and measure is a candidate for a state variable, such as its size, the number of its dendritic and axonal branches, its rate of energy consumption, the con-centrations of ions and molecules inside and around it, and the rates of transfer of those chemicals across various parts of the membrane (Figure 5). The most useful state variables for my purposes are derived from the electrical potentials that a neuron generates, either across the neural membrane (its trans-membrane potential) or in the tissue around it (its extracellular potential field). Recordings of these electrical potentials, which give estimates of the amount of energy being used by neurons, enable us to define one state variable for axons and another one for dendrites. They are significantly different from each other.

A neuron acts on another neuron by sending an electrical pulse to its dendrite by the synapse. The second neuron's dendrite responds to the pulse, not by immediately giving a pulse of its own, but by generating a dendritic wave of electrical current that flows to the cell body, where it appears as a postsynaptic potential. The axon expresses its state in the frequency of its action potentials (its pulse rate), whereas the dendrite expresses its state in the intensity of its synaptic current, (its wave amplitude). So the elementary forms of axonal and dendritic activity differ.

Because a neuron must stay active in order to stay healthy, even at rest the typical cortical neuron has a low pulse rate averaging about a pulse a second. As each pulse lasts only a thousandth of a second, the neuron is seldom in the pulse state, but the continual activity is essential to maintain its health. There is a corresponding irregular synaptic current in the dendrites to match the average pulse output of the neurons. These activities constitute the normal background state of neurons when brains are at rest or asleep. They can be suppressed by chemical anaesthetics, or by removing part of the brain and keeping it alive in a dish. Studies of neurons under such conditions can be misleading because the neurons are not healthy.

The significance of the differences between the axonal pulse and the dendritic wave lies in the differing nature of the tasks these two parts of the neuron perform. The dendrites integrate the pulse inputs they receive after they transform the pulses to waves, whereas the axons transmit the neuronal output as trains of pulses. The axonal pulse height is relatively fixed, so the magnitude of the output is conveyed by the pulse rate, or more specifically by the time intervals between pulses. The energy for the pulses is provided along the entire length of the axon, so there is no attenuation (reduction in pulse height) from the start of the axon to the ends of its branches, although there is a delay because the pulse takes a short time to travel along the axon. Most importantly, two or more pulses cannot coincide on the same axon, as the axon cannot generate another pulse immediately, or for a relative refractory period after it, during which the capacity to generate another pulse gradually returns. Men experience a similar refractory period after ejaculation. So, the axonal pulse train carries neuronal activity from one place to another with a delay but without attenuation, and even with amplification by the number of its branches, but with only one pulse at a time on each branch.

When the pulse reaches the synapse it releases its chemical neurotransmitter, which diffuses to the dendrite where it opens a switch on a battery in the membrane, so the dendritic current starts to flow. The dendritic current released by a pulse at a

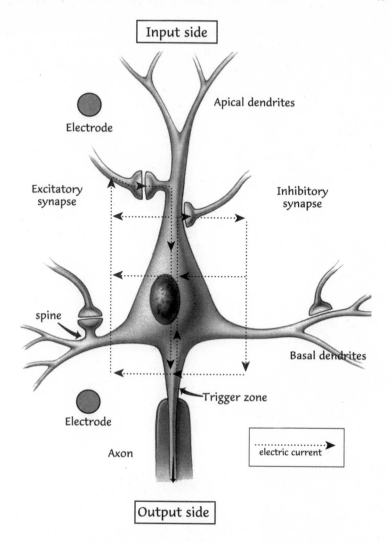

Figure 5 Typical neuron trees are connected by synapses. They have several dendrites to receive synaptic input, but only one widely branched axon to transmit output. Each synapse works like a switch on a battery that drives electric current. Input arriving on an axon switches the current on briefly. The current starts by flowing (dashed lines) inwardly at an excitatory synapse and outwardly at an inhibitory synapse. Output is initiated at the trigger zone, where excitatory current goes out and inhibitory current comes in. The current is the only way that synapses can act rapidly on the trigger zone. The sum of the microscopic loop currents there is the measure of dendritic input that determines the intensity of axon output. The microscopic current from each neuron sums with currents from other neurons around the neuropil. That sum causes a macroscopic potential difference, which we measure with a pair of extracellular electrodes as the electroencephalogram (EEG).

synapse rises rapidly during the thousandth of a second the pulse lasts and then returns more slowly to the resting level. It, too, has a fixed height and duration, but it differs from the pulse in that the wave of current can be superposed on top of the currents from other synapses, as well as under a continuous barrage, as in background activity. This capacity for the superposition of currents enables dendrites to integrate their input. The dendritic wave of the entire neuron varies continuously in proportion to the total number of pulses that all the dendrites receive.

We can show this by stimulating the incoming axons artificially with an electrical pulse from a pair of electrodes. The sum of the currents that a neuron generates in response to the electrical stimulus produces the postsynaptic potential, because current flows in one direction across the membrane at each synapse and in the other direction everywhere else (Figure 5), and as it flows across the membrane everywhere else, it causes an electrical potential difference to appear. This offers a good way for us to observe and measure its state variable in the wave mode. (Alternatively, a magnetoencephalogram, placed outside the body, can measure the magnetic field caused by the current in the dendritic shaft.) The strength of the postsynaptic potential decreases with the distance between the synapse and the cell body, so the contribution from a distant synapse is weaker at the cell body than that from a nearby synapse. This attenuation is compensated for by the larger surface area and the greater number of synapses on the distal dendrites, all connected through the cell body to the axon by the main dendritic shafts.

This dendritic loop current is the only way that synapses can rapidly send signals from the dendrites to the axon. Moreover, the action potential depends wholly on axonal loop current for its propagation. Therefore, eavesdropping on the electric and magnetic potential differences that accompany synaptic currents and action potentials provides our most direct means of knowing the active states of neurons. We pick up the messages that they themselves send and respond to.

Each neuron continually converts incoming pulses to waves, sums them, converts its integrated wave to a pulse train, and

Conversion Operations

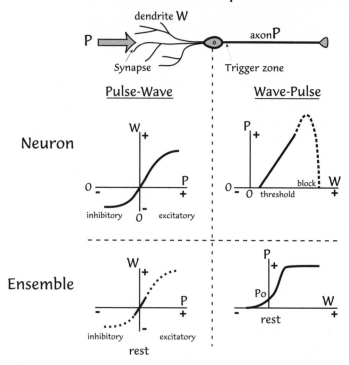

Figure 6 Dendrites make waves (W), whereas axons make pulses (P). Synapses convert pulses to waves, and trigger zones convert waves to pulses. In single neurons we measure microscopic pulse frequencies and wave amplitudes. In populations we measure macroscopic pulse and wave densities. We need a distinctive curve to represent each of the four conversions. All curves have upper and lower limits for output (vertical axes) with increasing excitatory and inhibitory input (horizontal axes), which we call bilateral saturation. We call an S-shaped curve a sigmoid. The steepness at each point of the curve measures the gain of the conversion. Where the slope goes flat with saturation, the gain goes to zero. Saturation guarantees stability, which is characteristic of homeostatic regulation. The steepest slope for pulse-to-wave conversions is in the centre at the rest point. In wave-to-pulse conversion for populations, the steepest slope is not at rest but on the excitatory side. We call this an asymmetric sigmoid; the asymmetry guarantees local instability. The middle section of each curve is almost linear, whereas the full curves are nonlinear. The nonlinearities make neural activity constructive and unpredictable.

transmits that train to all its axonal branches. To describe these conversions, we need quantitative descriptions (Figure 6). When a pulse arrives at a synapse, its chemical neurotransmitter switches on the synaptic battery and is then removed and degraded or recycled. When the battery is turned on at an excitatory synapse, the current flows inwardly at the synapse and outwardly everywhere else (Figure 5, left), but preferentially towards the cell body where all the dendritic currents are summed. The initial segment of the axon is also at the cell body, which has in its membrane the molecular machinery for generating pulses. This segment is called the trigger zone, and it is here that the outward-flowing current makes it more likely for a neuron below its pulse threshold to fire a pulse, and for the pulse rate in an already active neuron to increase.

An inhibitory synapse releases a different neurotransmitter, which turns on the membrane battery in the opposite direction. The current flows outwardly through the synapse and inwardly everywhere else (Figure 5, right). The same electrical properties hold for converging the current to the trigger zone, where it is subtracted from the excitatory current, so it decreases the firing probability of a neuron at rest, and decreases the pulse rate of an already firing neuron.

The process of transforming the dendritic wave into an axonal pulse train in the trigger zone is called wave–pulse conversion. As shown in Figure 6 (top right) for a single neuron, the pulse rate is directly proportional to the wave amplitude. The relation can be described by a straight line, but this linear relation holds only between the threshold, below which a pulse cannot occur, and some maximal excitation, above which the neuron fails to fire, because it has not yet recovered from the preceding pulse. Those limits are nonlinearities. The pulse–wave conversion at the synapse is also nearly linear in a broad middle range but saturates at both extremes. When the number of excitatory pulses is increased, the wave amplitude, which is the sum of the excitatory and inhibitory currents, increases as well, but with each new increment of increased input, the amount added on to the wave decreases. This diminishing return shows that the wave amplitude of a neuron cannot increase or decrease indefinitely. This relationship has the form of a sigmoid, or S-shape, curve (Figure 6, top left), which means that the neural activity is limited in both directions: it cannot increase or decrease indefinitely. These limits are responsible for keeping neural activity – and brain activity – within normal ranges. In other words, the state space of each neuron has resilient boundaries, because the closer a neuron gets, the harder it has to push to go further.

Because the current flows only in a closed loop, it flows first across the membrane at the synapse, then along the inside of the dendrite to the cell body, and finally in the other direction through the extracellular fluid from the trigger zone to the synapse, completing the circuit (Figure 5). The flow of the loop current inside the neuron is revealed by a change in the membrane potential, which we can measure with an electrode inside the cell body. This is how we evaluate the dendritic wave state variable of the single neuron. The flow of the same current outside the neuron is also revealed by an electric potential, but it is much smaller in amplitude. Although the current is the same, the resistance of the tissue outside the neuron is much lower than the resistance of the membrane. But there is an even more important difference. Whereas the path inside the dendrites is private for the neuron, the path outside is very public. The same path is shared for the loop currents of all the neurons in the neighbourhood, so that electrodes placed outside the neurons, as shown in Figure 5, measure the cortical potential that is established by the sum of the dendritic currents in the neighbourhood. The same currents produce the membrane and cortical potentials, but the two methods of observation and measurement, intracellular and extracellular recording, give two very different views of neural activity, one microscopic, the other macroscopic.

Now we have to consider how neurons make populations, and how we can measure their states. Neurons initially grow from embryonic cells that divide and multiply in very large numbers to give densely packed, nearly spherical cells. When the axons and dendrites begin to grow, they extend rapidly with prolific branching between the cell bodies. Many neurons die if they fail to make adequate connections. Even so, in the adult cortex, the density of cell bodies is so high that there are typically a million or more other neurons within the radius of the dendritic arbor of a given neuron. Although each neuron connects with only about one per cent of the neurons within its reach, there are still at least ten thousand input and ten thousand output connections for each neuron. This dense network of axons, dendrites, synapses and interconnected neurons, along with the blood vessels and the branches of supporting cells, called glia, forms the tissue we call neuropil (from the Greek *neuro* and *pilus*, meaning 'felt'). This is what the grey matter of the brain and spinal cord is made of. The neuropil of the cerebral cortex is distinguished by its architecture, in which the projection cells (also called pyramidal cells because of their shape) have their cell bodies in layers and their apical dendrites aligned perpendicular to the cortical surface (Figure 4).

The initial connections between neurons in embryonic cortex seem to form blindly, based on chance encounters between cells in the neuropil, as the axons and dendrites branch and extend. The strengths of connections are maintained by continuous activity at low levels, while the cortex waits for changes in synaptic strength to be made with learning and habitual use. In mature cortex are some basic patterns of connection, which we use to describe the dynamics of interactions. The input to one neuron from other neurons is convergence (Figure 7). The output from a single neuron has divergence to other neurons. Successive synaptic connections in series form chains. We say that axons that form nerves, tracts and bundles, and send their action potentials simultaneously side by side, transmit in parallel. Neurons that excite others and receive excitation from them in return form cooperative feedback networks, because they tend to act together; this is a form of positive feedback. Neurons that inhibit other neurons and, having shut down their neighbours, are then released from inhibition, form a competitive feedback circuit because some cells, being released, give yet more inhibition to their neighbourhood. This is also a form of positive feedback, because the initial trend that is set into action is maintained by the interaction. It contrasts with negative feedback, by which

Neural connections

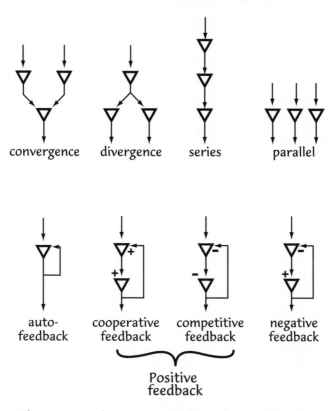

Figure 7 The connections between neurons that make networks and populations provide the material substrate of intentional behaviour. The basic kinds of forward and feedback connections are shown, where + indicates excitation and – indicates inhibition. Neurons do not excite or inhibit themselves synaptically (autofeedback) because input from their own output is only one among a million.

excitatory neurons arouse inhibitory interneurons and are then inhibited by them, so the direction of initial action is reversed by the feedback. This homeostatic feedback serves to keep things as they are.

We can observe these connection patterns in images of neurons that have been impregnated with heavy metals (Figure 4) in procedures called Golgi staining. They provide the elementary connection types for neural networks. But the images are misleading because, like the wires in electronic circuits, they do not move, whereas live dendrites wriggle like a bucket of worms, and also because less than 1 per cent of the neurons are visible in Golgi stains of cortical tissue. The images therefore give the illusion of sparse networks, whereas in fact the packing density of neurons is extraordinary, and no one neuron or small number of neurons can make another neuron fire or not fire. For the same reason, 'autofeedback' (Figure 7) does not occur, because the likelihood is one in a million that any connection received by a neuron comes from itself, and, even if it did, the neuron would be refractory because of its own output. It is important that the feedback connection types in Figure 7 also apply to masses of neurons in neuropil. Each neuron interacts directly with neurons in its neighbourhood, and indirectly by serial synapses, so the entire brain is reached within a few serial synapses from every neuron.

Not all neurons are interconnected by synaptic feedback. The groups of sensory neurons in the somatic, auditory, gustatory and olfactory systems transmit in parallel and with divergence but with virtually no feedback to each other. Each collection forms what I call an aggregate of neurons because they do not interact, and we will discuss them further in Chapter 4. But the cortical neurons, by virtue of their synaptic interactions, do form neural populations. The defining characteristic of the neural population is the sparse yet high density of synaptic interactions each neuron has with many others. We use microscopic pulse and wave state variables to describe the activity of the single neurons that contribute to the population, and macroscopic state variables to describe the collective activities to which the neurons give rise, also in the pulse and wave modes. We measure the microscopic state variables of neurons in time scales of a thousandth of a second and a spatial scale of thousandths of a millimetre, and we scale the macroscopic state variables of populations in scales of seconds and millimetres, because populations are larger and act more slowly than neurons.

Instead of using pulse frequency, we can describe the mass activity in a local neighbourhood in the brain by a pulse density.

We can observe the pulse density by recording from outside the cell the simultaneous firing of the pulses of many neurons in a neighbourhood. In the wave mode we observe the amplitude of the wave density by measuring the electrical potential difference between the surface and the depth of the cortex. This is given by the flow of the dendritic loop currents from the neurons in the local neighbourhood across the electrical resistance of the cortical tissue. The electrodes in Figure 5 towards the top and bottom of the left-hand side show how we measure this difference. The same current that controls the firings of the neurons gives us the EEG, which we mentioned earlier. We cannot distinguish the individual contributions, but we do not need to.

Just as a neuron can be described as a collection of membrane molecules and pores in axons and dendrites, a population is a collection of local neighbourhoods, each corresponding to what we commonly call a cortical column. Columns are not fixed anatomical structures, like nuclei in the brainstem, but dynamic patterns of activity, like clouds and vortices, with characteristic sizes and energy contents. The description of the macroscopic state in an area of cortex includes the amplitudes of the pulse and wave densities in the collection of columns that specify a spatial pattern in the two dimensions of the cortical surface.

Conversions of both pulses to waves and waves to pulses occur in each local neighbourhood. At the collective trigger zones, where wave density is converted to pulse density, the relation differs from that between dendritic wave amplitude and axonal pulse frequency in the single neuron; in other words, the macroscopic differs from the microscopic. At the microscopic level the wave–pulse relationship is linear between sharp limits of threshold and blockade, and the steepness can change rapidly over time, but at the macroscopic level the relation is nonlinear and does not change over time. Unlike in the single neuron, wave–pulse conversion in the population is a sigmoid curve (Figure 6, bottom right) that imposes limits. The resting level of pulse activity is low but not quite zero, because the neurons in cortical populations generate background activity by continually sending pulses to each other at random time intervals, whether or not there is sensory input or motor output.

As the wave density in a neighbourhood goes to the inhibitory side, the pulse density goes to zero with decreasing firing probability of the axons in that neighbourhood. At the other end of the curve, as wave density goes to the excitatory side, the trigger zones in the population encounter the refractory periods progressively, and pulse density approaches an upper limit, because neurons need to recover between pulses: as the neurons in a neighbourhood are excited to higher levels of activity, there is a corresponding increase in the number of cells still recovering from previous activity. The average pulse density in a population can never approach the peak pulse frequencies of single neurons, because the average includes the absolute and relative refractory periods, as well as the inactive periods intervening between successive pulses.

The pulse–wave conversion at the synapses in a local neighbourhood is also sigmoid (nonlinear) because the synapses in the dendrites cannot be driven too far outside their normal ranges. But the sigmoid curve in pulse–wave conversion at synapses is much wider than at trigger zones. The wave–pulse conversion always precedes the pulse–wave conversion and so it sets the boundaries. The limits at the trigger zones hold the activity of neighbourhoods in the centre of the dendritic sigmoid curve, where it is very nearly linear (Figure 6, bottom left). This finding greatly simplifies the description of populations. Because the wave–pulse conversion is nearly linear, we have only one main nonlinearity to be concerned with in describing the dynamics of neural populations. Moreover, it can stay fixed for long time periods, whereas the nonlinearities of single neurons vary rapidly, which greatly complicates the microscopic dynamics.

Neural populations are similar to macroscopic ensembles in many complex systems. There are four requirements for them to form: there must be many semi-autonomous, independent elements, such as neurons; each must have weak interactions with many others, so pair bonding is not crucial; the input–output relations of the elements must be nonlinear; and there must be a huge source of matter and energy, and a limitless sink for waste products and heat. Systems that meet this criterion are said to be open. Brains and their component neurons, particularly in cortex, meet all of these requirements, but they are not unique to brains. Macroscopic ensembles exist in many materials, at many scales in space and time, ranging from the chemical assemblies within single cells up to ecological networks, social organizations, weather systems such as hurricanes and tornadoes, and even galaxies. In each case, the behaviour of the microscopic elements or particles is constrained by the embedding ensemble, and microscopic behaviour cannot be understood except with reference to the macroscopic patterns of activity.

The formation of macroscopic states is the first step by which neurons, through their collective action, form activity patterns that transcend the cellular level and begin to approach the level of the organism. The process is non-local, in the sense that no one neuron takes command, nor is there any unique prescribed trajectory to be followed. Having attained through dendritic and axonal growth a certain density of anatomical connections (Figure 4), the neurons cease to act individually and start participating as part of a group, to which each contributes and from which each accepts direction. So, above a certain threshold of anatomical connection density, neurons in an aggregate (which are non-interactive) change their state to be the same neurons in a population (they are interactive). Their behaviour changes. This transformation of the neurons from one mode of existence to another is an example of the state transition. The activity level is now determined by the population, not by the individuals. This is the first building block of neurodynamics.

The threshold for the state transition is reached when each neuron receives from other neurons as many pulses as it gives to those in its neighbourhood. For example, in an excitatory aggregate below threshold, excitatory neurons excite each other in positive feedback (Figures 7 and 8, middle frame). So, when a neuron gives 100 pulses on average but receives only 80 pulses in return, then those 80 pulses next give only 64 pulses in return, and so on through successive cycles until the activity returns to zero. The ratio of 80/100, or 0.8, is called the gain of the loop. As the connection density continues to increase, each neuron receives 100 pulses for the 100 pulses it gives. This is the threshold for population formation. The gain is 100/100, unity.

Once it is activated, however briefly, the aggregate, now a population, continues its activity indefinitely without further input. When growth continues and each neuron receives 120 pulses for each 100 it gives, the gain of 1.2 exceeds unity, and the activity level can theoretically increase with each successive cycle around the loop from 120 to 144 and so on without limit, but in practice this does not happen because of saturation. The individual refractory periods determine the upper limit of the sigmoid curve for the population. Just like our amorous male lover, every neuron rests between pulses. The saturation effectively reduces the gain, until the gain returns to unity, and a non-zero steady state is reached. This contrasts with the zero steady state, in which the neurons all return to silence after perturbation. When they continually excite each other strongly enough, they cannot let each other remain silent, so they natter on. Yet, no matter how dense the synaptic connectivity may become by virtue of growth, the excitatory population always comes to a steady level of activity, with no need of inhibition to curb it. Once that steady level is reached, it can rebound from inhibition, as well as recover from excitation, when it is perturbed from outside. In other words, the population also is semi-autonomous.

As growth continues, the amplitude of the steady state increases proportionally, so that adults have stronger steady states than children. Other factors also come into play, including arousal, which we experience as hunger, thirst, sexual interest, curiosity and so on. The changes are accompanied by an increase in the steepness of the sigmoid curve of brain populations. It is regulated by neurochemicals secreted by brainstem nuclei under limbic control, so the steady states of excitatory populations can wax and wane with fluctuations in the intensity of intentional states.

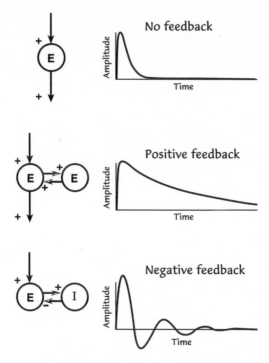

Figure 8 The forms of macroscopic responses of neuropil to a pulse input reveal the type and strength of an interaction. The strength is measured as the feedback gain; if it is zero (no feedback), the impulse response decays quickly (top trace). This is also the form of the classical microscopic postsynaptic potential of single neurons. When excitatory neurons (E) interact with each other (positive feedback) the response is prolonged (middle trace). If the gain is equal to one, the response to a pulse lasts indefinitely. If the gain exceeds one, the response increases until saturation brings a new steady state by a state transition. When excitatory neurons interact with inhibitory neurons (I) by negative feedback, the response oscillates (bottom trace). The stronger the gain is, the longer the oscillation lasts. In cortex, excitatory neurons outnumber inhibitory neurons by nearly ten to one, so most synapses are between excitatory neurons. This positive feedback is the source of 'spontaneous' background activity because the cells continually excite each other. The return to a resting point reveals a point attractor, so called because, within certain limits, the neuropil activity returns (is attracted) to that level regardless of the intensity of the perturbing input. These limits define what we call the basin of the attractor. The state transition from a point attractor at zero activity to a non-zero point attractor giving steady-state activity is the first of ten building blocks of the dynamics of intentionality.

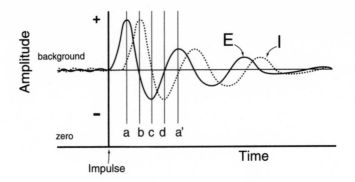

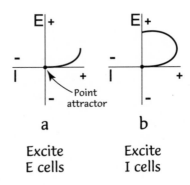

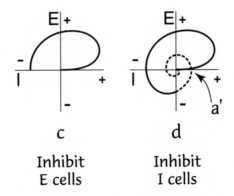

Figure 9 The upper graph illustrates the time sequence of events in negative feedback between excitatory (E) neurons and inhibitory (I) neurons that produces EEG oscillations. Oscillation occurs only in the presence of background activity, which comes from positive feedback among excitatory neurons that is stabilized by saturation. The four lower graphs show the state space of an area of cortex with a plot of the excitatory state variable on the horizontal axis (solid curve in the upper graph) and the inhibitory state variable (dashed curve above) on the vertical axis. The inward spiral to the resting point reveals a non-zero point attractor. Because of bilateral saturation (Figure 6), neuropil activity returns to that point, regardless of the intensity of the perturbing input, within limits that define the basin of the attractor. The emergence of oscillation through negative feedback is the second building block in the dynamics of intentionality.

An important property of this macroscopic state is its stability. We can demonstrate stability by perturbing the population with a sensory or electrical stimulus. An excitatory pulse increases the activity level briefly, but the population then returns to the steady-state level (Figure 8, middle). An inhibitory stimulus decreases the activity level briefly, but again it returns to the steady state. The population is said to have a point attractor, because the population returns (is attracted) to the same level after it is released from a wide range of intensity and duration of stimuli. The range of amplitudes that its pulse and wave densities can take defines the state space of the neural population. The portion of the state space to which the population can return in its steady state is called the basin of attraction, in analogy to a ball rolling to the lowest point of a bowl, no matter where in the bowl it is originally dropped.

One notable point that lies outside this basin is zero activity. If the population's activity is totally suppressed, so it becomes an aggregate, its activity does not resume unless at least one pulse is given to start it again. Normally this point is unstable because any pulse will always restart it, but zero activity can be made stable by deep anaesthesia, which suppresses background activity by setting the gain at the trigger zones to zero. We call this the open loop state, and the anaesthetic makes it stable under perturbation. In that condition, a stimulus in the form of a pulse elicits a brief response with the same form as postsynaptic (that is, dendritic) potentials of single neurons (Figure 8, top).

Engineers call this an impulse response; neurobiologists call it an evoked potential. It offers a valuable assay of stability.

In waking brains, the impulse responses are oscillatory, because the action of inhibitory neurons on the excitatory neurons that drive them provides negative feedback (Figure 7). Oscillations are so important that it is worth looking at how they emerge in cortex (Figure 8, bottom). Most neurobiologists think that single neurons fire spontaneously and rhythmically, like the heart does, but microscopic cortical neurons fire erratically like the crackle of lightning. The macroscopic interaction of each excitatory neuron with the neurons around it gives the stable point attractor, because the enormous number of action potentials are like the steady roar of heavy traffic. Each neuron may stay close to its threshold, waiting quietly until a throb in the noise pushes it to give a pulse, after which it returns to waiting again. This same principle of macroscopic regulation holds for oscillations. Each excitatory neuron is a member of an excitatory population that interacts with an inhibitory population. If such a mixed population is left to itself, it autonomously goes to a steady state because it has a point attractor. Its capacity for oscillation is revealed by giving an electrical shock to the axons that deliver its input. The shock is like striking a bell with a hammer: it rings at its characteristic frequency until the ringing decays to the steady state. The ringing in cortical activity is the evoked potential. Oscillation is the second of our building blocks.

In a graph showing how amplitude changes with time (Figure 9), the oscillations of both the excitatory and inhibitory populations have the same frequency and decay rate, but the inhibitory wave lags behind the excitatory wave by a quarter of a cycle. The reason for the lag can be seen in another view of the impulse response when it is plotted in the state space, where the excitatory amplitude is on the horizontal axis, the inhibitory amplitude is on the vertical axis, and time is shown by a point that goes anticlockwise around the centre of the space where the axes cross. The track of the point is shown by the solid curve. In Figure 9a, the incoming axons end on the excitatory neurons and excite them. In Figure 9b, the excitatory cells excite the inhibitory cells, which reach their peak of excitation a quarter of a cycle later than the peak of the excitatory cells' activity. At this time, the excitatory cells are already inhibited to their basal, resting level, but they overshoot under the continuing input from inhibitory cells. They reach a maximum of inhibition just as the inhibitory cells return to their basal level (Figure 9c). The inhibitory cells during this phase fail to receive the usual background excitation from the excitatory cells, so they undergo inhibition (Figure 9d). The release from the normal strength of inhibition means that the excitatory cells are ready to rebound, but only if they have a source of excitation.

They do. At this time (Figure 9a'), the response would terminate if there were no background activity, which comes from mutual excitation. When the excitatory cells are released from inhibition they are again free to respond to the background activity, and so give a new surge of excitation to the inhibitory population. This starts another cycle of oscillation but at lower amplitude, and it repeats until the ringing dies away. The frequency is somewhere between 20 and 100 cycles per second, which we call the gamma range, although it is commonly mislabelled '40 Hz'. Oscillations in this frequency range are familiar to everyone. Examples are the hum of electrical power stations, the chatter of car and motorcycle engines, and the purring of cats. The decay of oscillations as the evoked potential returns to the basal, resting level before the stimulus reveals the point attractor. This pattern occurs for a wide range of amplitudes of excitatory and inhibitory pulse inputs to the cortex, and this range defines the basin of the attractor. When the cortex is released from sustained input, it returns to the starting point, showing that the basal state is stable. The state designated by the point cannot be an attractor unless it is a stable state. We generally take it for granted that basal states are stable, and we use pulse driving to determine the degree of stability, which is equivalent to the size of the attractor basin.

We use the decay rate, which is the rate of return to the basal level, to measure the ratio of any peak to the preceding peak.

This ratio serves to evaluate the gain around the cortical negative feedback loop. The gain can be changed by a variety of manipulations. For example, suppose that the evoked potential from the cortex of an awake animal gives a gain of 0.8. If the animal is lightly anaesthetized, the decay rate increases and the gain decreases to 0.6 or less. Under deep anaesthesia that suppresses the background activity, the gain goes to zero in the open loop state (Figure 8, top). The evoked potential then ends (Figure 9b) because the output of the excitatory cells is suppressed by the anaesthetic. If the animal is given a drug that enhances the excitatory synapses, the oscillation is prolonged and the gain rises to 0.9 or higher. If the ratio and the gain exceed unity, so that each peak is larger than the one preceding it, then a state transition occurs because the population does not return to the point attractor. The oscillation grows until it encounters the nonlinear limitations, and there it stays. We call this steady-state oscillation a limit cycle. It is the third of our building blocks.

Just like the steady background of mutual excitation, the oscillation becomes semi-autonomous, self sustaining and self organized. It is a stable state because, whenever we give additional excitatory or inhibitory input, the oscillation is temporarily increased or decreased, but on release from input, the population returns to its basal oscillation. In other words, a stable limit cycle attractor is revealed (Figure 10, bottom). No matter where the population state variables are pushed to by input such as a pulse, whether inside or outside the dashed circle in Figure 10, the output returns to the circle after the input ends.

We have now come a long way towards understanding how neurons organize their activities to produce brain function. The important point here is that neurons form macroscopic entities by their interactions on a grand scale, in much the same way that molecules form liquids and people form societies. The way to give substance to this truism is to look at the differences between the activities of single neurons compared with those of populations. A good example is to watch the pulse trains of single neurons that are embedded in a population, which is

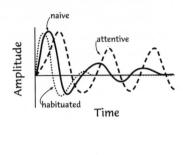

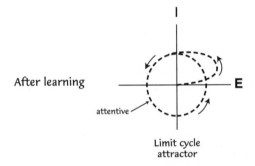

Before learning

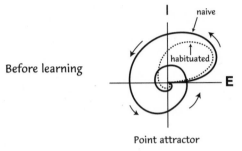

After learning

Figure 10 A state transition is required to go from the steady state of a point attractor to the sustained oscillation of a limit cycle attractor. This is illustrated by the learning-induced change in the impulse response. The evoked potential of the olfactory cortex before learning is shown by the solid trace. First an animal learns to ignore the evoking stimulus (habituation). This decreases the loop gain, so the cortex returns more quickly to its rest point (dotted trace). The cortex is stabilized with respect to that stimulus. It then learns to respond to the stimulus behaviourally (attention). This increases the loop gain and the oscillation persists (dashed trace). The cortex is therefore destabilized selectively with respect to that stimulus. The gain changes are due to synaptic modifications with learning. We call it a limit cycle attractor because, when the oscillating system is perturbed, it returns to the same pattern of oscillation after further excitation or inhibition over a wide range. That range defines the basin of the attractor. The state transition from a point attractor to a limit cycle attractor is the third building block of the self-organizing dynamics of intentionality.

governed by a limit cycle attractor. Typically, when the EEG wave of the population shows a regular oscillation with a peak of around 40 times a second, the single neurons fire once or a few times each second, and then erratically on one or a few peaks. Statistical analysis is required for us to see that these neurons are not only influenced by the oscillation, but are producing it. Their commitment to the whole is neither obvious nor compelling. The single neuron is largely autonomous, tending its own affairs, but the small part of its resources that it does devote to the whole is the measure of its significance for the work of the brain. Moreover, every neuron is always involved to some extent, and the nature of its participation changes with each state transition of the whole, as the cortex jumps from one point or limit cycle attractor to the next, and thereby from one task to the next.

State transitions in cortex can be induced by using drugs, which can also bring about behavioural transitions, such as putting an animal to sleep using an anaesthetic, or driving it into a frenzy with amphetamine. But these drug effects are not relevant to intentionality. Behavioural changes are germane, particularly in respect to the evoked potential. If an animal is trained to ignore the electrical stimulus used to evoke the potential wave, the animal habituates to the stimulus and the ratio of the oscillation decreases, showing that habituation decreases the gain selectively for that stimulus. The cortex undergoes a selective state transition that makes it more stable to that stimulus without impairing its responses to other stimuli (Figure 10, top).

However, if the animal is trained to respond to the stimulus when the trainer pairs it with reinforcement, such as by giving it food if it presses a switch whenever the stimulus is given, then the evoked potential shows prolonged oscillation that implies an increase in the gain. In other words, association learning increases the negative feedback gain, and that decreases cortical stability selectively to the conditioned stimulus (Figure 10, bottom). Can the gain ratio exceed one, with output amplitude exceeding input amplitude, so that a limit cycle attractor can be triggered by the learned stimulus? The evoked potential technique cannot answer this question, but other techniques using the EEG show that it can. The results, which are discussed in Chapter 4, indicate that each sensory cortex has not only zero (open loop) and non-zero (steady state) point attractors, but a collection of learned limit cycle attractors. Strictly speaking, they are not limit cycle attractors, but they are closely related. The state space of the cortex can therefore be said to comprise an attractor landscape with several adjoining basins of attraction, one for each class of learned stimuli. We describe the activity of a sensory cortex in a waking animal as an itinerant trajectory over its landscape, because the cortical EEG reveals a succession of momentary pauses in the basins of attractors, to which the cortex travels once a learned stimulus has arrived. The attractors are not shaped by the stimuli directly, but by previous experience with those stimuli, which includes preafferent signals and neuromodulators as well as sensory input. Together these modify the synaptic connectivity within the neuropil and thereby also the attractor landscape.

In summary, neurons act individually at the microscopic level to bring sensory input into the brain and spinal cord and to carry motor output to the muscles and glands. Neurons in the brain interact synaptically to create populations with macroscopic states, which constrain the activities of the neurons in accordance with local mean fields of intensity. Interaction by mutual excitation creates non-zero steady states that we see in the background activity of waking and sleeping brains. These stable operating points, called point attractors, provide the set points around which brain activity is stabilized. They are essential for the oscillations of excitatory and inhibitory neural populations that are synaptically coupled in negative feedback loops. In turn, stable oscillatory states are governed by limit cycle attractors. As we will see, the basic property of intentionality is to generate behaviour from within the brain, not merely to respond passively to stimuli. The positive and negative feedback loops of neural populations are responsible for this ability to create behaviour freshly with each new moment. The state transition between attractors is the way in which itinerant trajectories of brain activity arise, governing what we experience as habitual behaviours, and it is the landscape of attractors formed by learning that is responsible for reliable sequences of goal-directed behaviours. These attractors and behaviours are constructions by brains, not merely readouts of fixed action patterns. No two replications are identical: like handwritten signatures, they are easily recognized but are never twice exactly the same. We now turn to the details of how the constructions take place in sensory cortices, and look at the next four building blocks of neurodynamics.

Chapter 4

Sensation and perception

Along with other animals, we act in the world and then change ourselves in accordance with the impact the world has on our bodies following our actions. This is a circular process that can be said to have a motor output limb and a sensory input limb. Most biologists study the input limb in isolation as a linear chain of events. They initiate the chain by giving a stimulus to the body of an experimental subject. This is a reasonable simplification, because the time, place and manner of stimulation can be set by the researcher. The output limb is much more difficult to predict, measure and control, because the intentional actions initiated by the subjects come not when the biologists decide, but when the subjects do. Although we will first look at the input limb, ultimately I hope to put the output limb first, especially its originating process, intentionality.

The input limb has two main steps, sensation and perception, which are as different as night and day. The concepts and experimental methods used to understand the principles that govern sensation cannot be extended to explain perception. We will start by having a quick look at the basic properties that hold for all sensory systems. The main problem that each sensory path addresses is the generalization over equivalent sensory receptors. This problem arises because sense organs, such as the nose, eye and skin have immense numbers of receptor cells, which serve to optimize the capture of odorant molecules, photons, hairs moved by contact, and so on. These receptive surfaces are the interfaces between the finite body and the infinitely complex world. Repeatedly giving the same stimulus excites only a small fraction of the receptors on each trial, and the fraction is different on every trial. So how does the brain perceive it as the same stimulus? This quality of perception is what we mean by 'generalization over equivalent sensory receptors', 'stimulus constancy' and 'perceptual invariance'. We will use the neurodynamics discussed in Chapter 3 to discuss how brains solve the problem of perceptual invariance using the sensory cortices.

A typical sensory receptor has much the same structure as all other neurons. It has a cell body, from which long filaments usually extend in two directions. Its input end corresponds to a dendrite, which extends through some part of the body, such as the skin, muscles, joints or the inside of the nose. The body includes the brain and spinal cord, which also contain sensory receptors for light, stretch, temperature, hormones and the chemical properties of the blood, but not for pain. The output end of the receptor is an axon that extends into some part of the brain or spinal cord. The entire neuron is completely enclosed by its membrane. But a sensory receptor differs from other neurons in the specialization of the membrane in its dendrite-like end. Each receptor neuron has one of a broad variety of chemical structures in or around its membrane that gives it a particular affinity to selected chemical substances, as in olfaction and taste, or to selected forms of energy, such as mechanical force, vibration, heat, light and electric or magnetic potentials, as in hearing, vision and touch. Despite these variations, the input end works in the same way as the dendrites of other neurons. The chemical binding or absorption of energy switches on a membrane battery, releasing a loop current that flows inside the cell to the trigger zone at the start of the axon and outside to the synapse to complete the loop. The current initiates a train of action potentials, which propagate to the ends of the axon branches. The current strength and the frequency of the pulses are both proportional to the stimulus intensity.

Everyone agrees in referring to this short chain of transformations as transduction, but they interpret it differently. In the materialist view, the receptor extracts information from one of the forms of physical energy, and its axon carries this into the brain as an analogue quantity. In the cognitivist view, the axonal pulse train is a binary digit, a symbol that represents the physical form of the stimulus. In the pragmatist view, the axonal pulse train is simply a quantity of energy that is proportional to the input of energy from the environment at a point in the body. There is no extraction of information or meaning from the stimulus by the receptor, and the pulses certainly cannot represent it.

Each sensory receptor is truly microscopic. It works as one of an immense number of similar receptors, which function between the world and the brain in two-dimensional aggregates and transmit without synaptic interaction. The axonal pulse train transmitted by each neuron is therefore determined by the absorption of energy from the local intensity of a sensory stimulus. The selectivity of receptors and their restricted sensitivity to grades of input, such as colours in vision, frequencies in sound, and concentrations of chemicals, means that a sensory stimulus activates only a small fraction of the total number of receptors in each aggregate at each instant of exposure. That fraction forms a spatial pattern in the aggregate that is transmitted by axons in parallel into the brain and injected there as another spatial pattern.

This parallel transmission provides for topographic mapping of patterns from receptor aggregates to sensory brain areas. Because the receptor neurons do not interact among themselves, the spatial patterns they make in the aggregate and in their central targets take the form of microscopic points that are comparable to constellations of stars in the night sky, flashing with each pulse. Neurobiologists often restrict their test stimulus to one or a small subset of receptors by using a point of light, a pure tone, or a touch to a single hair, but even so the input yields a spatial pattern with a pulse rate that is forced high at one location and assumed to be zero everywhere else, although that assumption is seldom tested. We will examine olfactory perception in depth because it is the dominant sense in most animals, and in vertebrates it provides the prototype for perception through the other senses. It is also the simplest system, as it has the least preliminary processing, which occupies so much of the visual and auditory systems in the refinements of perceiving sights and sounds. It is anatomically closest to the limbic system and has the most direct access to the parts of the brain involved in the expression of emotions. And most significantly, the olfactory, visual, auditory and somatosensory systems, despite having substantial differences with respect to sensation, must have essentially the same mechanisms of perception, because the messages from all these different sensory systems are combined at some level in the brain to form unified multisensory perceptions.

The olfactory system exemplifies these mechanisms, starting with its receptor aggregate (Figure 11) that sends parallel axons in the primary olfactory nerve to the olfactory bulb. The axons form excitatory synapses onto the bulbar projection neurons, which send their axons to other parts of the forebrain through the lateral olfactory tract. Each inhalation brings odorants to the nose, exciting small subsets of the specialized receptors sensitive to those substances. There are about one hundred million receptors in the noses of many animals, and genetic studies show that there are a thousand types of receptor sensitivity profiles, giving about one hundred thousand of each kind of receptor. Only a small fraction of each kind, perhaps a few hundred or a few thousand, is excited on each sniff, so a sparse spatial pattern of pulses is sent to the bulb with each sniff of air coming with a specific odorant. However, many background odorants come too, so the sparse pattern is buried in a landslide of receptor action potentials. It is the job of the olfactory bulb to detect a desired pattern obscured by the massive amount of noise.

The large number and high density of receptors allows the nose to capture odorant molecules at very low concentrations but, because the airflow through the nose is turbulent, the inhaled air carries the molecules to a different set of receptors with each sniff. This means that the spatial pattern of receptor pulses differs for each sniff, even when the same odorant is inhaled repeatedly. This variability is well known in the other sensory modalities as well. For example, sounds change with the position of the ears, and the spatial pattern of excitation in the

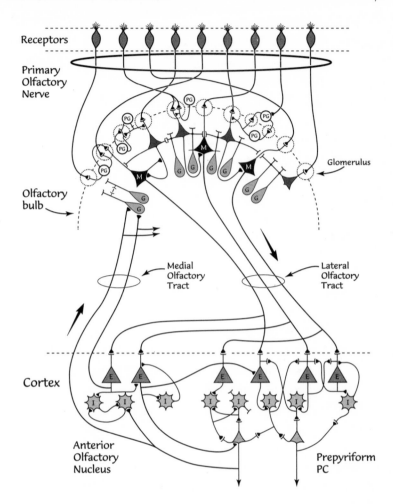

Figure 11 The olfactory system has four main parts: the receptor array in the nose, the olfactory bulb, the nucleus, and the cortex. Forward transmission from the receptors to the bulb is through the primary olfactory nerve, and from the bulb onward through the lateral olfactory tract. The nucleus and cortex feed back through the medial olfactory tract to the bulb, but not to the receptors. There are two populations of interneurons: the external interneurons (PG) provide the excitatory bias that is necessary for the background activity, whereas the internal interneurons (G) inhibit the projection cells (M) and, by negative feedback, provide the oscillations observed in the bulbar electroencephalogram (EEG). Negative feedback between projection neurons (E) and interneurons (I) within the nucleus and within the cortex also provides oscillations, but at different frequencies, owing to differences in internal feedback gains. These three parts of the central olfactory system cannot agree on a frequency, yet cannot ignore each other, so, as in a *ménage à trois,* they live in chaos. The genesis of chaotic background activity by feedback is the fourth building block of the dynamics of intentionality.

retina for a repeated stimulus changes as the direction of gaze shifts. Indeed, if a visual image is artificially fixed on the retina, it rapidly disappears from view, so that small changes in gaze are required for the image to be perceived.

Despite this variability, the behavioural responses are constant, including the verbal reports of humans and the actions of other animals. This invariance shows that the brain can generalize over the variations on repeated presentations and abstract some common properties. On this basis, we expect to find constancy in a spatial pattern of activity somewhere in the brain when the same odorant is presented repeatedly and is perceived as the same odour.

When I first began research into this problem, I expected that the patterns of microscopic pulses of bulbar neurons would be nearly as variable as the receptor-cell patterns were, because there is only a single synapse between the receptor axons and the bulbar projection neurons. I was not surprised when this turned out to be the case. In other words, there was no generalization by the microscopic bulbar neurons to the class of stimulus brought about by repeated presentations of the same odorant. But I was surprised to find a spatial pattern of bulbar activity that was nearly invariant over many trials with the same odorant. This pattern was in the bulbar EEG at the macroscopic level. Furthermore, the pattern covered the entire bulb, so that every neuron in the bulb was involved with every stimulus presentation. These properties held for the patterns that accompanied every learned odour, so I concluded that every neuron is involved with the perception of every odour.

This gives a very different picture of the transition from sensation to perception from the one generally advanced by neurobiologists and cognitivists, who hold that the information from an odorant is focused by the bulb into just a handful of neurons. Instead, my research shows that the brain generalizes by forming a macroscopic pattern of activity that includes the small number of neurons bringing the activity into the brain, and a lot more neurons besides. And it happens at the very site where the axons come into the brain and form the first serial synapse in the brain, in the olfactory bulb.

This conclusion is so important that I want to describe how my students and I made the observations and interpreted the measurements, and go on to describe the relevant macroscopic properties in detail. The generalization pattern in the EEGs of the bulb appeared in the high-frequency oscillations that we identify as the gamma range. Remarkably, the oscillations of the dendritic potential have the same waveform over the whole bulb. This must mean that the common wave is due to the interactions of neurons throughout the entire bulb, because there is no pathway from the receptors or from inside the brain that can force all the neurons to oscillate in the same way over such a wide range of high frequencies. The patterns are therefore created by the neurons within the bulbar population, not imposed from outside. Pattern genesis is a common phenomenon in chemical and physical systems. For example, a clear sky can produce puffy clouds in a matter of minutes. It should come as no surprise that this microscopic process works in sensory cortices, and the only reason it has not been observed before is that no one has predicted what to look for in the gamma range.

To make these observations, we put some rabbits to sleep using a chemical anaesthetic, surgically exposed the sensory areas, attached arrays of electrodes to the skull, and closed the lesion carefully to avoid infection and minimize the rabbits' discomfort. During surgery we fixed a rectangular array of 64 electrodes, spaced half a millimetre apart to give a 4 millimetre by 4 millimetre window on the bulb. With the help of veterinarians, we nursed our rabbits to full recovery from the surgery. We then familiarized them with our recording apparatus and connected the implanted electrodes to a set of amplifiers and a computer to display the EEGs.

Our recording systems allow us to detect the patterns of activity covering the entire bulb, even though our window covers only a fraction of it. We know from other experiments that the bulb works as a unit, and we know that, even if most of the bulb has been surgically removed, animals can still discriminate

odours, regardless of which part remains. Olfactory discrimination needs only a few connections from the receptors
into the bulb and from the bulb into the olfactory cortex. Because
all parts of the bulb seem to be equivalent in this way, we could
place our array at the most convenient place on the bulb. Again,
this is very different from the materialist and cognitivist predictions, that responses to each odorant would be restricted to
one small part of the bulb, like each key on a computer keyboard.

Four findings are particularly important. First, the bulbar
neuropil shows continual background activity with aperiodic,
and therefore unpredictable, waveforms. This background is
maintained by the mutual excitation among the projection
neurons (M in Figure 11) and external interneurons. This self-
stabilizing background activity is the fourth building block of
neurodynamics.

Second, with each inhalation there is a burst of activity that
ends after exhalation. The burst is everywhere in our window,
and we have shown it is all over the entire bulb at the same
instantaneous frequency (Figure 12), even though that frequency
keeps changing within and between bursts. The oscillations are
due to the negative feedback interactions when the excitatory
projection neurons interact with the inhibitory internal interneurons. The shared frequency is due to the widespread interconnections between the projection neurons, by which every
excitatory neuron reaches every other in a few synapses.

Third, the common wave has a different amplitude at each
location in the bulb, so the wave serves as a carrier wave in the
gamma range, with a spatial pattern of amplitude modulation
(AM) throughout the bulb. I call the wave a carrier because the
waveform is the same everywhere but its amplitude varies. The
AM pattern is the fifth building block of brain dynamics. By
measuring it in the EEG we can estimate the output of the bulb,
because the dendritic currents that determine the EEG also
determine the spatial patterns of the internal interneurons,
which in turn determine the pulse density function of the projection cells. We measure the amplitude of the common wave at
each of the electrodes, and display the 64 amplitudes in contour

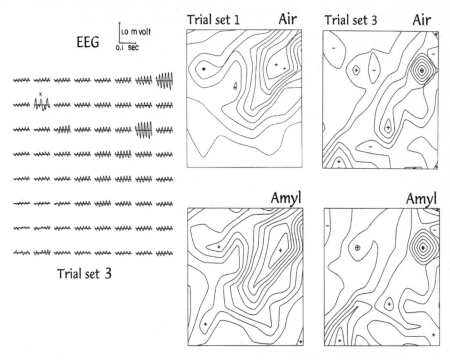

Figure 12 An 8×8 array of electrodes makes a 4×4 millimetre window onto the bulbar surface. The 64 traces of EEG contain short episodes of oscillation during each inhalation, called bursts. Each burst has the same chaotic waveform everywhere in the window and throughout the bulb. (The cross marks one channel in which I recorded an EEG from the bulb instead an EEG from the olfactory cortex in order to show a difference.) Each trial set shows the pattern before the stimulus ('Air') and during the stimulus ('Amyl'). The bulbar wave with the same form has a different amplitude at each location, which makes it the carrier of a spatial amplitude modulation (AM) pattern. This is the fifth building block of intentional dynamics. AM patterns change with learning and carry the contents of brain activity, which are the first stages of meanings, not only in olfaction but in all the primary sensory cortices. The carrier oscillations are often called '40 Hz', but gamma activity is a more accurate term because the frequencies vary over a range from 20 to 100 Hz or more in the same and different species. The four examples of AM patterns use contour plots to show the peaks and valleys of wave amplitude. Note that the AM patterns for both 'Air' and 'Amyl' change from trial set 1 to trial set 3, even though the odorants were not changed. From Freeman and Schneider (1982).

plots of the high and low amplitudes of activity in the bulb like hills and valleys (Figure 12, top four frames). Each contour plot gives us a simple way of representing the state of the bulb for other people. A sequence of plots reveals the state transitions that occur with successive inhalations (Figure 13, top). We classify EEG patterns with respect to odorants by using the AM patterns, such as those shown in the contour plots. We find that each recording channel contributes equally to the classifications of the AM patterns. No channel is any more or less important than any other. From our statistical sampling, we infer that every neuron participates in every discrimination, whether it is firing rapidly or slowly. Every pattern must have dark as well as light, and it is a mistake to assume that a neuron that is not firing in response to a stimulus is not part of a pattern: it may be silent because that is the role that is assigned to it by the macroscopic state of the bulb.

Fourth, we find that each rabbit has an AM pattern like a signature that, although it is never the same time, we can easily discriminate from the patterns of other rabbits. Each AM pattern is as unique for each rabbit as the individual history of the animal, and as the shape of its body and the colour patterns of its fur.

These findings raise the question of how the individual bulbar bursts (Figure 13) form? We know that input from olfactory receptors is required, because the bursts disappear if the nostrils are closed and breathing is through the mouth. The mechanism is based in the sigmoid curve we saw in Figure 6 (bottom right), which governs wave–pulse conversion at the trigger zones of neural populations. A graph from our experiments of the steepness of the sigmoid curve shows how much the pulse output changes for a given change in wave input. In other words, it depicts the nonlinear gain that determines how strongly the bulbar populations interact at each level of wave density. This graph shows that the excitation of the bulb by receptor input increases its wave activity, and the input also increases the gain, which measures the strength of the synaptic actions of the neurons onto each other. The higher the gain, the more prolonged

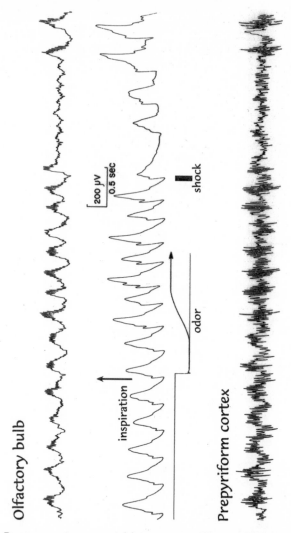

Figure 13 Bursts occur in sequential frames, as in a film. In olfaction, pulse densities in the lateral olfactory tract carry the AM patterns from the bulb to the olfactory nucleus and cortex and the entorhinal cortex. The bursts are triggered by inhalations because excitatory input increases the loop gain. Excitation pushes the system to a steeper part of the asymmetric sigmoid curve (Figure 6, lower left curve). Input that an animal has learned to identify can thereby selectively induce a state transition in sensory cortex. This input-dependent gain is the sixth building block of the dynamics of intentionality. The example shows EEGs from the bulb and cortex (upper and lower EEGs) after the rabbit had learned to sniff whenever it perceived an odour of banana oil (or amyl acetate, as in Figure 12), which it had learned would be followed by a brief electric shock that made it pay attention. The increase in rate and depth of breathing after the odorant arrived (middle trace from a device to measure respiration) shows its sniff. From Freeman and Schneider (1982).

are the oscillations. When the gain is increased enough, as we saw in Chapter 3, the oscillations start to explode, not die away. This is how the bulb is destabilized by inhalation. Input drives the bulb from its resting state and holds it in the burst state until exhalation, when the bulb is allowed to return to rest. These state transitions into and out of a burst are the crucial events that start and finish the first full step of perception in the olfactory bulb. The destabilization by input-dependent gain is the sixth building block of brain dynamics.

Instances of the sigmoid curve and its slope, the nonlinear gain, differ by only one parameter, which depends on whether the rabbits are asleep, anaesthetized, awake but inactive, or aroused and active. The nonlinear gain increases with arousal, as the more excited an animal becomes, the steeper is the sigmoid curve, and the more likely it is that input can destabilize the bulb. This explains why bursts seldom occur in animals that are not aroused, whether or not odorants are inhaled. In a sense, the bulb is turned on and made receptive by arousal, which is governed by the limbic system that controls the release of neuromodulator chemicals secreted by brainstem nuclei, in particular histamine, so the work of perception can be done.

The burst visible in the EEG shows that the bulb switches between two states. It is in a receiving state before each burst, and in a transmitting state within each burst, precisely as a single neuron switches between the states of getting and giving pulses. Before the state transition upon each inhalation, the bulbar neurons respond mostly to the input, but in the burst they respond mostly to each other. The bulb keeps an open door up to the state transition, but then the door is shut and the AM pattern is determined by the synaptic connections in the bulbar neuropil, rather than by the stimulus. During the bursts, the bulb transmits its AM patterns to other parts of the brain, and between them it receives both sensory input and preafferent corollary discharges.

How do spatial AM patterns differ between odorants? Materialists and cognitivists argue that the input from a sniff starts a spatial AM pattern of oscillation in the bulb that is maintained by reverberation in a limit cycle, like the ringing of a bell when it is struck, as we saw in Chapter 3. They account for the variations between the AM patterns within each cluster by the differences in patterns of receptor activation that are due to turbulence in the nose. According to their hypothesis, the brain would have to store, accumulate and average sets of AM patterns in a training period, and then retrieve the average pattern as a standard against which to compare all new incoming patterns during a test period, not only with one average AM pattern but with all other average patterns to find the best match.

My data show that brains do not have the neural machinery to perform these engineering operations, and if they did, they wouldn't have the time needed to run them. Specifically, I show that, even with fixed experimental conditions and invariant stimuli, the constancy of the pattern for each class of odorant holds for only a few days. The general rule is that slow changes in AM patterns take place over days and weeks, at a rate comparable to the growth of hair and nails. The changes appear to depend in part on the steady growth of axons and dendrites in the neuropil, and on the deletion, relocation and new formation of synapses. On top of these relatively slow changes, which we call perceptual drift, are dramatic changes that occur when the animals are exposed to odorants paired with a reinforcement, such as a mild electric shock to the skin, or food or water given to a hungry or thirsty animal.

Odour-specific AM patterns form only when we ask our rabbits to discriminate between odours. Typically, we offer either of two odorants, which we call conditioned stimuli (CS). One of the two, a CS+, is paired with a reinforcement, and the other, a CS−, is not. With reinforcement, a previously unimportant CS becomes meaningful to a rabbit, because it can predict and avoid a disagreeable experience, or seek a pleasurable one. Our rabbits give a conditioned response (CR) only to the CS+. The four frames in Figure 12 show how AM pattern changes with learning. The top left frame shows the average AM pattern in the control period before the CS+ was given. The bottom left frame shows the different AM pattern found after the rabbit had learned to respond to the CS+. We recorded the bursts after the CS+ began, but before the CR began. In this experiment, the control with its background odorants is equivalent to the CS–. We expected that the AM patterns with the CS+ and CS– would differ, and they did. But we did not expect what happened next: both patterns changed. The right frames show the control and CS+ patterns two weeks later. The stimuli and the behaviours were the same, but the AM patterns were different. We find that the AM patterns lack invariance with respect to unchanging stimuli.

Another example of the lack of invariance, in Figure 14, shows the results of serial conditioning. We familiarized our animals with the experimental apparatus, which in itself was a learning experience, and trained them serially to respond to sawdust, amyl acetate, butyric acid and finally sawdust again. Their AM patterns changed with each new odorant. On returning to the first odorant, the sawdust, their AM patterns were different from those recorded on the first exposure. So the AM patterns are dependent on context, history and significance – in a word, meaning – and this is the seventh building block of neurodynamics.

The most dramatic example of how learning affects AM patterns came about when we reversed the reinforcement between CS+ and CS–. We trained thirsty rabbits to lick a CS+ paired with water, and merely to sniff to a CS– without water. Then we switched the reward from the first odorant to the second one, and just as quickly the animals learned to lick after the second and merely to sniff after the first. These were the same chemicals and the same motor patterns, yet all three AM patterns changed. The amounts of change were small, but they significantly exceeded the amount of change predicted from measurements of daily drift.

We showed that changes in the AM pattern were due to the modification of synapses in the neuropil. We did this by training cats and rats to respond to an electrical pulse given to the lateral olfactory tract and measuring the evoked potentials in the cortex and the bulb before and after the animals had learned to respond to the pulse as a CS+. The change in waveform (Figure 10) is due

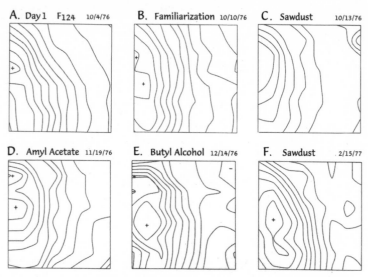

Figure 14 The bulbar amplitude modulation AM patterns are found in the gamma range of the EEG. They change whenever an animal learns to respond to a new odorant, because the CS+ (see text) is paired with a reward or a punishment. I expected, when I gave again an odorant already learned (here sawdust), that the old AM pattern would reappear, but it did not. A new AM pattern formed, and all other existing patterns also changed. Another example of this variation of pattern with a fixed stimulus is in the change between the 'Air' (control) patterns in sessions 1 and 3 in Figure 12. These findings show that the structures of the AM patterns depend on the history embedded in the neuropil by synaptic modifications during learning, and not on the individual stimuli. They reflect generalization over learned classes of inputs. Because of the contributions from past experience, they are aspects of the meanings of the stimuli, holding only in the animal that has constructed them. This embodiment of meaning in AM patterns is the seventh building block in the dynamics of intentionality. From Freeman and Schneider (1982).

to an increase in the gain of the synapses that interconnect the projection neurons in the bulb and the cortex (Figure 11). There is no change in the gains of the incoming synapses from the receptors to the projection cells, where most researchers expect to find changes with learning. The increased synaptic gain with associative learning destabilizes the neuropil only to those stimuli that have acquired meaning through reinforcement. The change with learning is highly selective, based on the stimuli given during the training period.

The outcome is very different if reinforcement is not paired with an unfamiliar stimulus. The first event when a new olfactory stimulus arrives is the failure of a burst to occur. The animal expects some odorant that it already knows, including the familiar background. The new odour means that the background fails to occur as expected. This failure is a signal for animals, because it leads to an orienting response, in which the animals turn their heads and eyes and sniff in search of an unexpected, unknown odorant. Burst suppression seems to happen when the background is so contaminated with a new odorant that the destabilized bulb cannot reach a basin of attraction and make an AM pattern. This is a state of 'I don't know what it is, but it may be important'. If the new odorant is reinforced, then a new AM pattern is formed, and the existing AM patterns are jostled and slightly modified. If it is not reinforced, then both the EEG response and the orienting reflex disappear, and no new AM patterns form. This is called habituation. It is an automatic local process that incorporates unidentified stimuli into the background. Screening unidentified, unwanted, irrelevant input is a vital and continuous task for all primary sensory cortices. Receptors do not and cannot perform this task, because they do not have access to the sensory patterns. They contribute only their own pulses to the patterns, rather like points in a pointillist painting.

These are highly significant phenomena. They show that AM patterns in the bulb are selective and specific for learned odorants, but that they lack invariance with respect to the chemical structure of the odorants. Each AM pattern depends on the history of exposure not merely to one odorant, but to every odorant. Moreover, each new learned odorant and new contingency of reinforcement leads to a change in the entire ensemble of AM patterns. The ensemble is based on dendritic and axonal growth and the modifications of synapses with learning, and the bulb requires continuing interaction through behaviour and the totality of sensory flow for the expression of its contents in AM patterns.

To use the language of dynamics developed in Chapter 3, we say there is a single large attractor for the olfactory system, which has multiple wings that form an 'attractor landscape'. The system has a preferred basal AM pattern between inhalations, which is governed by one wing of the large attractor. When an inhalation brings in background air, the bulb transits to the basin of another attractor wing that gives the control AM pattern, and it returns to the basal wing after release during exhalation. This attractor landscape contains all the learned states as wings of the olfactory attractor, each of which is accessed when the appropriate stimulus is presented. Each attractor has its own basin of attraction, which was shaped by the class of stimuli the animals received during training. No matter where in each basin a stimulus puts the bulb, the bulb goes to the attractor of that basin, accomplishing generalization to the class. A new odorant is learned by adding a new attractor with its basin, but, unlike a fixed computer memory, an attractor landscape is flexible. When a new class is learned, the synaptic modifications in the neuropil jostle the existing basins of the packed landscape, as the connections within the neuropil form a seamless tissue. This is known as attractor crowding. No basin is independent of the others.

The synaptic mechanism needed to account for generalization with a learned stimulus is provided by the increased interaction among bulbar neurons after the state transition induced by the input. This cannot happen in the receptor layer, because those neurons do not interact. The change with learning is that synapses are strengthened, but only between those bulbar excitatory neurons that are driven by examples of CS+ receptor input. When receptor input from an odorant CS+ comes to pairs of projection cells simultaneously, so they are active at the same time, and when it is quickly followed by reinforcement, then the synapses linking those pairs are strengthened. If there is no reinforcement on interspersed trials with an odorant CS-, or merely with the background, then the connections are weakened by habituation in the cortex, not in the receptor layer. During the trials needed for training to each new odorant, each sniff excites a different selection of the receptors sensitive to the CS+, and the corresponding pairs of projection cells they excite. Each trial adds new pairs, linked in a network to those both previously and presently active.

This criterion of shared activity for increasing the synaptic gain is known as the Hebb rule, and results in the formation of what we call a Hebbian nerve-cell assembly. The strengthened excitatory connections support the sweep of activation through the entire assembly when any subset of its members receives input. This is not pattern completion, because there is no defined external pattern to be filled in; it is only the odorant molecules falling randomly on point receptors. This is a case of generalization over equivalent stimuli. The cumulative synaptic modifications form the basin of attraction that leads to an AM pattern. Any new combination of previously stimulated receptors can then access the attractor, whether or not it has ever occurred during the learning period, because that combination puts the bulb into the learned basin of attraction. This is the synaptic mechanism of generalization.

This mechanism, which occurs in the olfactory bulb during learning to identify an unfamiliar odour under reinforcement, brings us to the most elementary step in the way brains generate meaning. It is the way in which neurons in the bulb make themselves similar to the form of a stimulus in the world, and so perform the process of assimilation. Like Thomas Aquinas and Jean Piaget, I consider assimilation to be fundamental to my theory of meaning. It begins when the chemical odorant attaches to and activates pairs of receptors simultaneously. The receptor cells do not need to be identical, and often they are not, because they can respond to different kinds of other odorants, but the stimulus does have the capacity to excite both of them. The axons of these receptor cells send action potentials to a pair of projection cells, which are excited, and which excite each other. If the pair of projection cells receives the neuromodulators that are released by reinforcement (we will discuss this further in Chapter 5), under the Hebb rule their synaptic connections are strengthened. If either one is excited in the future, they will excite each other preferentially. In this sharing in activity, they have become similar to the pair of receptors in the body, which in turn have an affinity to the stimulus in the world.

Of course, many pairs of receptors are activated together on each inhalation, and different but overlapping distributions of pairs are activated together on repeated sniffs. The form of the nerve-cell assembly that grows over several trials with reinforcement assimilates to the form of the odorant, although the similarity is not to the chemical structure. Rather, it is the match between that chemical structure and the spatial distribution in the nose of receptors that have an affinity for that structure. Each receptor acts at a point in space, and each projection cell integrates over the domain of its dendritic arbor, but no one cell carries a spatial pattern. The form of the input from the world is assimilated by the form of the AM pattern in the brain through successive steps of creation by the brain, leading from microscopic to macroscopic scales. This process shows why the form of an input is not transferred or injected as information into the meaning structure of a brain. Instead, the brain creates a simulacrum, or copy, that is compatible with the history and goals of the organism. This is the basic cellular process of assimilation, the enactment of the unidirectional relation of the self to the world. The constructions revealed by the AM patterns result from what Aquinas called the imagination, and what I call the nonlinear dynamics of neuron populations, and they relate to the meanings of the stimuli, not the unique and evanescent details of each injection of sensory input.

Each AM pattern is a macroscopic state variable that is carried by the pulse densities of the populations of bulbar neurons. The physicist Hermann Haken calls that state variable an 'order parameter' that 'enslaves' the members. The macroscopic field constrains and shapes the pulse probabilities of the component neurons. But it has a weak influence over an immense number of neurons, so it is not easily seen in the firing patterns of single neurons unless the patterns are averaged. The same neurons also participate in pulse patterns that are imposed by the inputs. The microscopic pulse frequency pattern evoked by the learned specific or background stimulus coexists with the macroscopic pulse density pattern that is established by each state transition.

These two patterns of pulses are transmitted simultaneously by the projection-cell axons to their targets. If there were a topographic mapping from the bulb by the tract to the cortex, as there is from the receptors to the bulb in the primary olfactory nerve, then the microscopic pattern would be registered in the cortex, as it is in the bulb by the transmission of sensory input from receptors through the nerve. But the tract is not organized that way. It is a divergent–convergent path (Figure 15). Each projection cell scatters its output broadly over its targets. Conversely, each neuron in the cortex receives from a wide distribution of projection cells, so it performs a spatial integration over the bulbar output.

The effect of this spatial integration is to enhance the AM pattern, because it has the same waveform everywhere, and the pulse trains of all projection cells carrying that waveform can be added without cancellation. But the stimulus-evoked activity is spatially incoherent, so it is diminished by smoothing. I call this process the 'brain laundry'. The activity of the brain is a cauldron of neural pulses, and at each transmission the pathway must clean the signal and wash out the noise. The spatial integration done by the tract defines the macroscopic AM pattern given to the rest of the forebrain as the signal from the bulb, and it rejects the microscopic activity driven by the stimulus as noise. The sum of local currents gives the EEG by a form of spatial integration (Figure 5), so the surface EEG gives a much better measure of the cortical signal than the microscopic pulses do. This is the main reason why the EEG is so valuable: it shows us which fraction of the bulbar output is actually being sent to the rest of the brain. Pulse recordings do not show that.

We have dealt with the mechanism of generalization, but we need to address another level of perceptual constancy, namely the stimulus–response invariance with which we began our inquiry. The AM patterns are never the same twice with the same odorant, yet the same CR follows the same CS. This is because the populations of neurons in the cortex also form nerve-cell assemblies, at the same time that the bulbar assemblies form during learning. Just as a bulbar assembly provides generalization

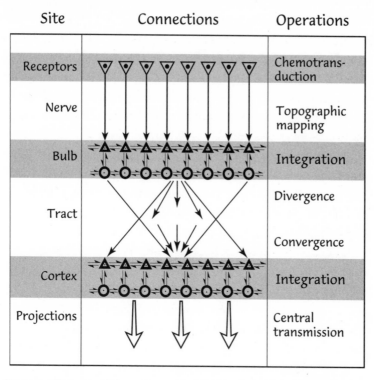

Site	Connections	Operations
Receptors		Chemotransduction
Nerve		Topographic mapping
Bulb		Integration
Tract		Divergence
		Convergence
Cortex		Integration
Projections		Central transmission

Figure 15 The axons in the primary olfactory nerve carry the microscopic patterns of sensory input from the receptors in the nose to the projection neurons in the bulb. These axons run in parallel, and we call this kind of transmission topographic mapping. It preserves specific details of the input, particularly in regard to spatial relations. The tract that carries output of the bulb to the cortex has no topographic order. Instead, it is a divergent–convergent pathway (Figure 7) because each bulbar neuron spreads its output broadly, and each cortical neuron collects input from a wide distribution of bulbar neurons. The tract smoothes the pulse patterns sent from the bulb to the cortex. The smoothing attenuates the microscopic sensory-driven activity coming from the bulb but enhances the macroscopic self-organized AM pattern, which carries the meaning. As a result, all that the brain receives from the bulb is what the bulb has itself constructed. This is the eighth building block of intentional dynamics. It provides the neural mechanism for the unidirectionality of intention identified by Thomas Aquinas. Adapted from Freeman (1992).

over a class of receptor inputs, a cortical assembly provides generalization over equivalent bulbar AM patterns, even in the face of drift and the secondary changes due to attractor crowding, when new stimuli or new schedules of reinforcement are added. If those changes are so great that the bulbar input fails to access the basin of an appropriate olfactory attractor, the animal fails to construct an appropriate action. It makes a mistake and suffers loss of an expected reward or is otherwise punished, so it continues to learn until the landscape of the basins of attraction has been properly updated to the present circumstances. The circumstances change in any case, because environmental change is inevitable.

Generalization and perceptual constancy are all the more remarkable considering that the neural activity through which they are achieved is so erratic and seemingly disorganized. To understand this, we need to be clear about the difference between chaos and noise. The background activity of the bulb and other areas of cortex consists of the continuous firing of neurons. The pulses occur irregularly and unpredictably with respect to their own history and the pulse trains of their neighbours. At the microscopic level, they lack temporal and spatial patterns, such as periodic oscillations. When we play a recording of this activity on a loudspeaker, it sounds just like a radio when we are looking for a station, and that is why we call it noise. But this noise provides an important component of the background when it is viewed as a macroscopic order parameter, because the interaction of excitatory neurons by their uncorrelated action potentials produces the excitatory bias that makes oscillations possible. Although the microscopic action potentials are not synchronized, the macroscopic bulbar EEG waves are the same everywhere, even between bursts. The constraint that all of the neurons maintain on each other by their interaction produces the macroscopic order parameter that, according to Haken, enslaves them. Physicists say that their degrees of freedom are reduced. Their autonomy is limited. The EEG is not periodic, like the tick of a clock, but irregular, and so it looks like noise. The microscopic activity really is noise, but the macroscopic activity is chaos. The main difference is that noise cannot be easily stopped and started, whereas chaos can be switched on and off like a light, because it manifests a constraint on the noise.

The olfactory system sustains its own chaotic activity even after we isolate it surgically from the rest of the brain and measure its EEGs. The waveforms are indistinguishable from those of the intact brain, except that state transitions with sleeping, arousal and associative learning under reinforcement do not occur. The EEGs before and after the surgery have statistical regularities that show the stability of the olfactory basal state, which is governed by a chaotic attractor. The stability of this background state can be seen when the system is perturbed, either with electrical or odorant inputs, or by briefly changing its synaptic gains using short-acting drugs, and observing that the bulb returns to the same state after recovery. In a graph of its trajectory, unlike the circle shown in Figure 10 for a limit cycle attractor, the chaotic attractor has the appearance of a bowl of spaghetti, owing to the unpredictable twists and turns of the trajectory folding back on itself. The pictures are not particularly informative, so let's not bother looking at one.

This background chaotic attractor is not a property of the bulb, but of the entire olfactory system. Although its microscopic components (the neurons) and its mesoscopic modules (bulb, anterior olfactory nucleus, and prepyriform cortex) can in some circumstances generate chaotic activity, in their normal ranges they do not. Each module has only a point attractor and a limit cycle attractor with its characteristic frequency. The chaotic activity results from the coupling of these three modules (Figure 11). The three frequencies differ, so that the system cannot settle on any one or them. Yet, by being coupled by an excitatory path in the forward direction, and by both excitatory and inhibitory paths in the feedback direction, the modules cannot escape one another. Negative feedback acts continually to curb the amplitude of activity, keeping it within predictable bounds. Positive excitatory feedback prevents the system from settling to a point attractor. The three modules create what I refer to as a neural *ménage à trois*, because that is an intuitively appealing description of a chaotic situation.

Many other parts of the brain have chaotic attractors and multiple wings, and the stability of their EEGs shows that they are exceedingly robust. Chaotic dynamics provides a basal state with ideal properties. The olfactory system cannot stay at a point attractor, because that can occur only when the neurons are silent, and inactive neurons atrophy and die. Their basal activity cannot be periodic, because sooner or later they would entrain into synchronous firing that is rigid and hard to change. This does occur in the highly synchronized discharges seen in epilepsy and in Parkinson's disease, but those are incompatible with intentional behaviour. The basal chaotic attractor keeps the system in a high-level state of readiness to move in any direction. We say that the system is close to the boundary of its basin of attraction, so that a state transition to a neighbouring basin can take place with a small but significant perturbation. There is actually a sequence of basins through which the system passes. Such a trajectory reflects chaotic itinerancy. Again this is an analogy to the travelling salesperson going from one town to another, who repeats the pathway but differently on each return. Just as there are preferred AM patterns, there are preferred sequences of AM patterns that are accessed by preferred trajectories from one attractor to another through the landscape. Like the habits of humans and their pathways through familiar territories, the trajectories are inviting, broken in, and well-used curves across an attractor landscape in brain state space.

Yet unpredictability is inherent in chaotic trajectories, and introduces flexibility and creativity in the construction with each new state transition. Chaos generates the disorder needed for creating new trials in trial-and-error learning, and for creating new basins in assimilating new stimuli. Its high-frequency oscillations maximize the likelihood of firing coincidences, which are required during the process of Hebbian learning. As a result, brains are drenched in chaos. It gives an optimal balance between flexibility and stability, adaptiveness and dependability.

So far we have focused on perception in the olfactory system, but what about the other senses? By measuring the EEGs of the primary sensory neocortices of rabbits trained to respond to light, sound or tactile stimuli, we know that these neocortical populations have essentially the same chaotic dynamics as the olfactory system, based in the same essential properties of neuropil. Neurons in large numbers are interconnected diffusely each with many others, yet still sparsely, owing to the high packing density. The mix of excitatory and inhibitory neurons gives rise by negative feedback to oscillations, which are continuous and aperiodic, indicating that they are governed by chaotic attractors. Each area has a common carrier waveform, which supports AM patterns, and these patterns change in the same manner as in olfaction when the animals are trained to discriminate between conditioned stimuli. The AM patterns occur in staccato fashion, resembling frames in a movie film. They show the same lack of invariance with respect to the stimuli under reversal of reinforcement, and the same tendency to long-term drift.

The importance of these findings lies in the demonstration that all the central sensory systems use essentially the same dynamics and the same signalling. Such conformance is required at some level so the cortical messages can be assembled into multisensory perceptions in the limbic system. The details of the visual, auditory and somatic inputs must be washed away, leaving only the meanings of stimuli as the signals to be combined. This is the eighth building block of neurodynamics.

By way of summarizing, we will see how the data on the AM patterns can be interpreted in different ways, depending on your choice of philosophical premises. According to the materialist view, these AM patterns reflect information processing. In this reasoning, for example by Stephen Grossberg, an odorant stimulus delivers information to the receptors, which process it by transducing it to action potentials. These pulses are transmitted to the bulb, where the information is bound into patterns and held, while it is being relayed by the tract to the cortex. The information stored in the cortex from previous stimuli is retrieved and sent back to the bulb (Figure 11), where a comparison is made by correlation of the newly received AM pattern with each of a collection of retrieved AM patterns. Grossberg uses the sigmoid curve to optimize the signal-to-noise ratio. The classification process is completed when the best match is found to identify an odorant. That best AM pattern is sent to other parts of the brain, where it serves to select and guide a fixed action pattern as a response to the stimulus. This provides a powerful neural network for use in engineering, but it does not correspond well with findings from brain imaging, such as the AM patterns in the EEG.

In the cognitivist view, each AM pattern represents an odorant. It is a symbol that signifies the presence of a source of food or danger. The receptor action potentials represent the features of the odorant, and the process by which the bulbar action potentials are brought into synchrony through their synaptic interactions to represent an odour is feature binding. The integration of the features by a higher-order neuron makes it fire, and its activity represents the object that has the features. So-called 'situated cognitivists' distinguish between external representations, such as contextual odours of places that are associated with food and that signify the location and kind of food, and internal representations, which are the AM patterns, the inner tokens made by brains from external representations in accordance with the logical rules of deduction and association. This approach cannot deal with the lack of invariance of AM patterns with respect to stimuli.

According to the pragmatist view, the AM patterns are an early stage in the construction of meaning. They correspond to the 'affordances' advanced by J. J. Gibson in ecological psychology, by which an animal 'in-forms' itself as to what to do with or about an odorant, such as whether to eat the food or run from the predator giving the odorant information. They cannot be representations of odorants, because it is impossible to match them either with stimuli or with pulse patterns from receptor activation that convey stimuli to the cortex. It is also impossible to predict in detail the patterns that are constructed in the bulb from the patterns of receptor activation, because the constructions are by chaotic dynamics. They cannot be information, because that is discarded in the spatial integration performed by divergent–convergent pathways. They are unique to the history of the individual, arising out of the past experience that shaped the synaptic connections in the bulbar neuropil. They reveal the wings of attractors that are selected by the sensory pulses, each having a crater in the olfactory attractor landscape.

The bulb sends both the macroscopic, self-organized AM patterns and the microscopic, stimulus-induced pulse patterns to other parts of the brain, but only the AM patterns really have an effect on the other parts to trigger their self-organizing responses, because the tract performs spatial integration, not topographic mapping. There is anatomical and physiological evidence for similar divergent–convergent projections from all the sensory cortices. These findings have a profound implication. The only patterns that are integrated into the activities of the brain areas to which the sensory cortices transmit their outputs are those patterns they have constructed within themselves. In colloquial terms, the ingredients received by brains from their sensory cortices with which to make meanings are produced by the cortices. They are not direct transcriptions or impressions from the environment inside or outside the body. All that brains can know has been synthesized within themselves, in the form of hypotheses about the world and the outcomes of their own tests of the hypotheses, success or failure, and the manner of failure. This is the neurobiological basis for the solipsistic isolation that separates the qualia of each person from the experiences of everyone else, and it is the neurophysiological confirmation of the inductive principle of unidirectionality that originated with Aquinas.

Chapter 5 | **Emotion and Intentional Action**

Imagine waking in winter when it is still dark outside and finding yourself staring disagreeably at your reflection in the bathroom mirror, unable to remember getting out of bed. Now picture yourself walking into the kitchen and starting the habitual work of making breakfast. You fill the pot with water and open the coffee jar. Empty! Someone forgot to fill it. Imagine your feelings of frustration, anger and resentment. Now fully alert, you start planning what to do about this disappointment. This is the essence of intentionality, a mixture of habitual routines and innovations surrounding an implicit goal and, quintessentially, a strong reaction to a stimulus that isn't there. This is the only time in this little sequence when you become fully aware. What is going on in your brain, and who or what is calling the shots?

Our actions emerge through a continuous loop that we can divide into three stages. The first stage is the emergence and elaboration within our brains of goals concerning future states, towards which we will direct our actions. The goals are in nested layers, ranging from what we do in the next few seconds to our ultimate survival and enjoyment of life. The second stage of the loop involves acting and receiving the sensory consequences of actions and constructing their meanings. In the third stage, we modify our brains by learning, which guides each successive emergent pattern. These three stages are accompanied by dynamic processes in the brain and body that prepare the body for forthcoming actions and enable it to carry them out. My view is that we observe and experience these preparations as emotions, although emotions are not as simple as that.

Our hearts pound, our palms sweat, and our stomachs churn when we face stressful situations that require us to do something, especially to avoid giving in to panic. But we also have to consider the popular idea of emotions as expressions of power in human affairs, which many people think is something that can be tapped for the energy needed to engage in creative activity, but also as something to be afraid of, because there is a risk of losing control. The world's literature is filled with plays, poems, novels, clinical treatises and philosophical tracts about emotions taking over, and they are a focus of scientific research into the origins of behaviour. I will settle for describing emotions from the perspective of their relations to the biology of intentionality, not as powers in the physical sense, but as manifestations of brain dynamics. In this way I hope to clarify some of the issues concerning the control and use of emotions as essential aspects of, but subordinate to, intentionality, perception and the construction of meaning.

The departure from a state of unflappable calm is aptly named: e(x)motion, meaning outward movement or intent. An emotional state may not be revealed in immediate overt actions, but it certainly implies the high probability that actions will soon be directed by an individual into the world. Such states are easily recognized and explained as intentional in many situations, but in others they seem to boil up spontaneously and illogically within an individual in defiance of conscious intent. They may be in apparent contradiction to sensory triggers that seem trivial, contrary or insufficient to account for the intensity of the actions. Yet they may have an internal logic that comes to light only after probing into and reflecting on the history of the individual. What is emotion, and why do we so often, wrongly I think, contrast it with logic and reason?

We can begin to make sense of emotions by identifying them with the intention to act, and then to note their increasing levels of complexity. At their most basic, we see the 'stretching forth' of intentionality in simple animals as they prepare to attack in order to get food, territory or resources for reproduction, or to avoid impending harm and find shelter. The important characteristics are that the actions well up from within the organism, and that they are directed toward some future state, which is being determined by the animal in accordance with its perceptions of its evolving condition and history. These simple forms of emotions are called 'motivation' or 'drive' by behaviourists. Those are poor terms, because they confuse intentional states with biological reasons, such as the need for food and water. They treat behaviours as genetically fixed action patterns that are triggered by stimuli from the environment, and they cause psychologists to look for 'drive centres' in brains, like batteries in toys that are controlled by external switches. They cannot explain phenomena such as curiosity, self improvement, and self sacrifice. Motivation and drive are also commonly conflated with arousal, which is a nonspecific increase in the sensitivity of the nervous system that need not be locked into any incipient action, and that may or may not follow a triggering stimulus. In other words, the concepts of motivation, drive and arousal lack either or both of the two key properties of emotions – endogenous origin and intentionality – and they beg the question of intent.

At a more physiological level, emotions include the expression of internal states of the brain. Behaviours that evolve through interactions with the world towards the future state of an organism predictably require adaptations of the body to support the intentional motor activity. These preparations consist of taking an appropriate postural stance with the musculoskeletal system, such as the readiness of a cat waiting to pounce on a mouse, and mobilizing the metabolic energy required for muscular actions. They include the cardiovascular, respiratory and endocrine systems, which are called upon to increase cardiac output to supply oxygen and nutrients to the muscles, and to remove the waste products of energy expenditure. It is the directedness of these preparations in positioning the body, heightening respiration, twitching the tail, erecting the hair, dilating the pupils, and so on, that reveals to observers the increasing likelihood of approach, attack or escape.

Among social animals that live in packs and tribes, these preparatory changes in the bodies of humans and other animals have become, through evolutionary adaptation, as shown by Charles Darwin, external representations of internal states of meaning and intended action. The displays, such as panting, pawing, stomping the ground, erecting the hair or sexual organs, or moving the face or limbs, serve as signals from an animal to represent its state to others around it. For transmission of such signals to succeed, a basis must have been formed through previous experience of social interactions. That prior agreement can have been made only by repeated actions coordinated among the members of the society, particularly by the play of juveniles, such as mock combat under parental supervision. This aspect of emotions as social communications is dealt with in Chapter 7.

At a more complex level, many of us think that emotions are experiences. They are the feelings or qualia that accompany emergent actions and address the anticipated futures of gain or loss in our attachments to others, our livelihood and safety, and the perceived possibility or impossibility of changing the world to our liking or advantage. We know them as joy, grief, fear, rage, hope and despair. The biological mechanisms of these qualia remain controversial.

In the materialist tradition, physiologist Walter Cannon identified them with the activity of neurons in the head ganglion of the autonomic nervous system, which is in the hypothalamus and sends neural messages to the sensory cortices. Neuroendocrinologists, such as Jaak Panksepp and Candace Pert identify them as operators composed of specific neurohormones that are released into the forebrain by specialized neurons in the brainstem. In the pragmatist tradition, psychologist William James proposed that the feelings are sensed after the fact, so to speak, through the changes in our bodies caused by the activity of the autonomic nervous system, such as our gasping and sighing, our bristling hairs, the pounding of our pulse, or our flushed face. The missing pieces in his puzzle were the internal messages conveyed by preafference. Materialists think the opposite: that these feelings are secondary side effects, while what you really feel are the messages your neurohormones give directly to the cortex and basal ganglia to shape the activity patterns forming in your brain, even though it is commonly and wrongly believed that you cannot feel stimuli given directly to your brain. Cognitivists have mostly stayed out of this debate, perhaps because a machine doesn't have emotions, and, like Mr Spock and Data, of Star Trek, that's cool. But some cognitivists would like to program emotions into their devices if they could figure out what they are and what on earth they are for. Pragmatists see the emotions as integral parts of the interaction between our selves and our social environments, including our own bodies. Through these bodily processes, in conjunction with preafference, we become aware of our emotional states, and, through the same processes as signals, our friends and enemies become aware of our states at the same time or even before we do. These perceptions of our states and actions, and of the states and actions of those important to us, shape our beliefs about our own state and next action. We will look at this again in Chapter 6.

The most complex level of emotions involves social evaluation and assignment of responsibility for actions taken. In the classical Platonic view, reason is contrasted with emotion. Actions that conform to social standards of considerate, productive behaviour are said to be rational, whereas actions that appear to lack the prior logical analysis we call premeditation, and that bring unwanted damage to oneself and others in the community, are said to be emotional. In my view, both kinds of actions are emotional and intentional, in that both emerge from within the individual and are directed to short- or long-term goals, but clearly they are different. The biological basis for that difference lies in the self-organizing properties of the brain, through which the chaos that engenders actions is constrained, and the actions are deferred by cooperation among the diverse parts of the brain. We experience that process as consciousness, and will examine it further in Chapter 7.

The core question here is the problem I raised in Chapter 2: how do intentional behaviours, all of which are emotional, emerge through the self organization of neural activity in even the most simple brains? I described the basic architecture of the simplest living vertebrate forebrain in Chapter 1, in order to introduce the simplest architecture of intentional action. That same architecture holds in the human brain, although it is obscured by other structures that have been elaborated by evolution. I will try to highlight the differences in interpretation of the basic architecture between the materialist and cognitivist views of the brain as an input-dependent processor of information and representations (Figure 16), and the pragmatist view of the brain as a semi-autonomous generator of goal-directed behaviours (Figure 17).

Materialists and cognitivists assign the starting point for analysis to the sensory receptors in the skin (as shown by the asterisk in Figure 16), eyes, ears or other points at which information from the world is transduced from energy to action potentials. Bundles of axons serve as channels to carry the information to the brainstem, where it is processed through nuclear relays and converged into the thalamus, which is a central sensory clearing house at the top of the brainstem. The information is already subdivided and classified by the receptors in respect to its features, such as colour, motion or tonal modulation. The thalamus sorts this classified information for transmission to small areas within each of the primary sensory cortices that are specialized to deal with their designated features. Because most of the channels dealt with by researchers form topographic maps with axons in parallel, they say that the information is topographically mapped from the sensory receptors in each sense organ into each of the small cortical areas. These researchers view the thalamus as acting like a postmaster to deliver the bits of information to destinations that have already been assigned by the sensory receptors. Within the thalamus, each relay nucleus inhibits the other nuclei. The nucleus that is most strongly excited suppresses the others around it. These others, being inhibited, fail to inhibit the excited nucleus, so it is more likely to transmit. Cognitivists call this form of interaction 'winner-takes-all'. They think that stimulus salience selects information for transmission to the cortex by con-

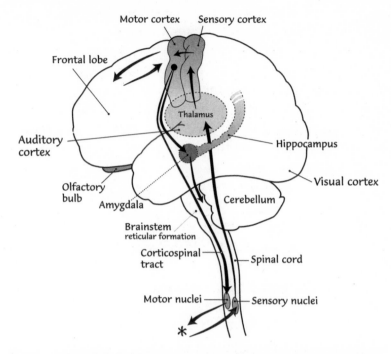

Figure 16 Materialists and cognitivists view perception as a passive process that begins when a stimulus (shown by the asterisk) gives information that is transduced by receptors into a burst of neural activity, which cascades through the brainstem and thalamus into a sensory cortex. Information processing then binds the activity of feature-detector neurons into the representation of an object. This is either stored in a local network of neurons or kept active and compared with other representations of previous stimuli that were stored and are now retrieved. That with the best match is sent by stages to the frontal lobes, where a decision is made to select an appropriate response. The motor cortex sends a command through the brainstem and spinal cord to the muscles. There are several noteworthy side loops. One upward loop is through the reticular formation in the brainstem and thalamus that produces arousal and selective attention. Another is through the cerebellum that fine tunes the behaviour. A downward loop is through the amygdala, which provides emotional tones from its repertoire of fixed action patterns and its controls on the secretion of emotionally specific neurohormones in the brainstem.

trolling attention. The hinge that squeaks the loudest gets the oil. Materialists and cognitivists both believe that when sensory input excites receptor neurons, their pulses represent primitive elements of sensation, or features. The primary sensory cortex combines these representations of features into representations of objects, and transmits them to adjacent association areas; for example, a combination of lines and colours might make up a face, a set of phonemes might form a sentence, and a sequence of joint angles and tissue pressures might represent a gesture. They believe that representations of objects are transmitted from the association cortices to the frontal lobes, where objects are abstracted into concepts to which meanings and value are attached. Somehow, in these chains of reaction, a sensation becomes a perception, but they haven't been able to show where that happens, or in what way a perception differs from a sensation, or where the information in a perception changes into the information in a command for a behaviour.

Parts of the frontal lobes seem well situated to carry out specific behaviours because they contain the motor cortices (Figure 16), whose neurons send their axons directly into the brainstem and spinal cord, where they connect to pools of motor neurons that stimulate specific groups of muscles. According to cognitivists, just as the neurons in the skin and soft tissues send information to the sensory cortex in an orderly way that forms a map of the body, the upper motor neurons from the motor cortex in the frontal lobe form a topographic map of the parts of the body that are controlled by the brain. Working backwards from the muscles in Figure 16, the final central relays provided by the lower motor neurons in the spinal cord and brainstem are driven by networks of neurons in the basal ganglia, which include part of the thalamus. At the crest of the chain is the motor cortex in the frontal lobe, with its map of the musculoskeletal system. The motor cortex in turn is controlled by premotor and supplementary motor areas that lie progressively forwards in the frontal lobes. Cognitivists view the frontal lobes as the site of selection and organization of motor activity. The motor maps are like piano keyboards, played by object detectors that ultimately derive from the sensory input.

These pathways for the integration of sensory information about objects and the formulation of motor commands may sound complicated, but the interpretations are based on straightforward engineering concepts. These concepts are supported by measurements of anatomical pathways in brains that have been

fixed, cut and stained, and by recording the pulse trains of cortical
neurons, mostly in response to artificial stimulus patterns given
to animals immobilized by anaesthetics. However the same
experiments done by some researchers, such as Moshe Abeles
and Miguel Nicolelis and their colleagues, but performed in
awake and behaving animals, show that stimuli activate neurons
that are widely dispersed, noisy and not restricted to rigid maps.
Furthermore, attempts to apply cognitive rules lead to intractable problems. For example, the thalamic winner-takes-all mechanism fails to account for expectancy, in which attention is
directed toward a stimulus that is not yet present. The corti-
cocortical pathways that link the primary sensory cortices to
the frontal lobes are well documented, but no one knows how the
features in the small specialized maps are combined to represent
objects, or even how an object is defined. How are elements
called 'primitives' combined to make a chair and a table, rather
than a combined chairtable? The binding problem is unsolved.
On the motor side, complete destruction of the motor cortex
interferes with finely controlled movements such as dancing
and playing the piano, but it does not otherwise interfere with
intention or the desire to dance and play.

In the cognitive view, the role of the limbic system is under-
played and seems mysterious, although it is known to be
involved with, maybe even required for, spatial navigation, the
enrichment of motor responses by emotions, and the formation
of explicit memories, as Larry Squire calls them to distinguish
them from implicit memories that are not readily accessible to
awareness. The neural mechanisms by which the limbic system
performs these functions are bundled into 'higher functions' to
be analysed after the problems of cognition have been solved. At
best, cognitivists propose a side channel through the amygdala,
which taps into primitive fixed action patterns and attaches
appropriate emotional modulations to cognitively driven behaviour. Lamentably, olfaction does not fit within cognitivists' interpretations and is either ignored or treated as a special case that
sheds no light on vision or audition.

While pragmatists have little agreement with cognitivists,

they do accept the materialist view of the anatomical organizations of the primary sensory and motor systems and their
functions under anaesthesia, as outlined above, but they assign
the starting point for the analysis of waking behaviour to the
brain. I assign it to the limbic system, not the sensory receptors
(asterisk in Figure 17). The consequences of this change in perspective are enormous. In particular, the pivotal roles of the
thalamus and the frontal lobes are reassigned to the limbic
system.

In simpler vertebrates, the limbic system comprises the entire
forebrain (Figure 3). The various goal-directed activities of these
free-ranging animals support the assertion that they have limited
forms of intentionality. In the human brain, the vast enlargement
of the neocortical lobes makes it difficult to see that the limbic
components have not only persisted, but have become enlarged
(Figure 17). For example, the hippocampus is still part of the
surface of each cerebral hemisphere, but the folding and twisting
of the hemisphere during its embryological growth buries it like
fingertips in a fist, so in humans it seems to be deep inside the
medial temporal lobe in the base of the brain (Figure 1). As
described by Pierre Gloor, it is only one of many modules that
make up the limbic system, but its central location, characteristic architecture, and long phylogenetic history make it a
focus for us to understand limbic dynamics. In metaphorical
terms, it is more like the hub of a spider web than the memory
bank or central processor of a computer.

In the salamander, the hippocampus receives input directly
from the primary sensory areas, whereas in humans and other
mammals there is a collection of intervening cortical areas dominated by the entorhinal cortex. It is the main source of input to
the hippocampus, and it is also the main target for hippocampal
output, so the two parts constantly interact. The most remarkable property of the entorhinal cortex is that it interacts with so
many other parts of the brain. It receives and combines input
from all the primary sensory areas in each cerebral hemisphere,
and it sends its output back again to all of them (Figure 17).
This reciprocal interaction in mammalian brains goes through

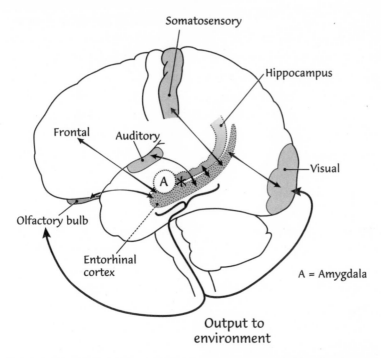

Output to
environment

Figure 17 Pragmatists view perception as an active process, holding that humans and other animals maintain a stance of attention and expectation. This stance embodies a hypothesis that is initiated by intentional dynamics in the limbic system, indicated by the asterisk and that is transmitted by corollary discharge to all the sensory cortices in the process of preafference. The arrival of stimuli confirms or denies the hypothesis. The hypothesis is tested by state transitions giving AM patterns that converge into the limbic system (into the entorhinal cortex in mammals). A new hypothesis forms, which presages one of a range of possible actions, each with its corollary discharge. The focus of intention is in the limbic system, not in the thalamus or frontal lobe, because the hippocampus has the neural machinery for directing intentional action through space–time. Every sensory module must have a mechanism for organizing its patterns of meaning in space–time. It must either have its own or share one mechanism after fusion of the multimodal patterns. Evolution has selected the parsimonious solution of time sharing. This does not preclude direct exchanges between sensory modules, but it indicates the unique importance of multisensory convergence into the entorhinal cortex, which is the ninth building block of the dynamics of intentionality.

multiple relays, which are identified by materialists as important stages for information processing from the visual, auditory and somatosensory cortices, and from the frontal lobes serving social interactions and long-term planning. Materialists also point to large pathways that support interactions between pairs of primary sensory areas, either directly or through thalamic relays, which they believe are the main basis for cognitive function. Pragmatists believe that these pathways help to shape what I call global activity patterns, which occupy the entire forebrain, but that the most significant aspect of limbic architecture is the multisensory convergence in the entorhinal cortex, followed by spatial localization of events and temporal sequencing of them in the hippocampus, which is required by other areas to form multisensory perceptions, or Gestalts, and to learn, remember and recall them.

The limbic space–time loop in Figure 18 is embedded in a set of nested loops. These loops have been deliberately simplified by the lumping together of many subsidiary components and lesser loops, in order to show the forest, not the trees. The space–time loop has been placed at the core because of two outstanding properties. First, the hippocampus has been shown experimentally to be deeply involved in the orientation of behaviour in space–time. Everyone agrees that intentional acts take place in space through time. The space is the personal realm in which the animal has moved in previous explorations and in which it now continues to move towards its immediate goals. The time is the personal lapse that every movement in space requires, and that orders each sequence of past, present and expected states. It makes architectural sense to find this space–time register located just after the multisensory integration, and before the entry into the motor systems. Neurobiologists find neurons in the hippocampus that fire pulses whenever an animal is in a particular place in its field of action. They refer to these neurons as place cells. Cognitivists believe that an aggregate of place cells in the hippocampus forms a cognitive map (a term introduced by psychologist Edward Tolman in 1950), which works like a memory bank to store spatial information in an atlas to represent the world within each animal. Pragmatists deny that there is any representation like a map, a look-up table, or a fixed memory store. Instead, they hold that the hippocampal neuropil maintains a field of synaptic connections among its neurons, and that this field continually directs behaviour by the interactions of the limbic system with the sensory cortices in the brain, as the animal moves from place to place through its environment.

This difference between the views of cognitivist and the pragmatist is subtle but important. Pragmatists find two ways in which we and other animals orient ourselves in space. One way is by a sense of direction around us with respect to prominent landmarks, such as the flow of a river or the location of a high building or hill. The other way is by remembering sequences of locations, as when we follow street signs in getting from a hotel to a bus station, provided we have done it before and can remember the chain of landmarks. Psychologist Lucia Jacobs has found evidence for these two mechanisms in different parts of the hippocampus of rodents that hide nuts in the autumn to find in winter. Jacobs finds that directional orientation is better developed in males, but that place sequencing is done better by females. She also finds that the part of the hippocampus that has the place cells enlarges in the autumn when the rodents are collecting and storing nuts, whereas it shrinks in the winter, when they are finding them. These anatomical changes are consistent with the widely held view that the hippocampus is required to form explicit memories and store them in other parts of the brain, but that it is not needed to recreate and use these memories during recall.

A similar view of spatial orientation without a map is advanced by engineers such as Jun Tani, Rodney Brooks, Andy Clark and Horst Hendriks-Jansen, who are building semi-autonomous machines that explore their environments and, in the process, learn to avoid obstacles such as walls, furniture and people. What they learn is not stored as a cognitive map in the archival sense used by cognitivists, but as switches in the machines that are set by learning, and that promote a direction of movement appropriate for each location in the learned space currently occupied. That is, the switches support interaction between the device and its environment by shaping specific actions in specific locations. We often navigate in this way when we walk or drive through a city that has become familiar through habitual visits, in contrast to stopping to consult a map of the city. Some people have the high-level ability to create symbols to make and read maps, but many do not, and we cannot infer that animals do, even in a metaphorical sense.

The second salient property of this space–time loop between the entorhinal and hippocampal cortices is that their neural populations have the same and similar kinds of interconnections and interactive dynamics as those in the primary sensory cortices. This means we can describe them using the same concepts and vocabulary that we used in Chapters 3 and 4. The EEGs generated by these structures have similar waveforms in time and space, and they show similar kinds of change with behaviourally related brain states as those displayed by the sensory cortices. My hypothesis is that the limbic populations, which comprise what I have schematized as the space–time loop, construct and maintain an attractor landscape. The basins of its multiple attractors formed by learning determine sequences of spatial AM patterns, such as those shown in Figure 14, that are achieved by repeated state transitions. The basins of its attractors determine the sequences of spatial AM patterns by repeated state transitions in chaotic itinerancy.

Each itinerant step is a global state transition, and such steps occur several times each second, which is comparable to what we experience as jumps in trains of thought. The underlying frames of local AM patterns occur up to ten times faster, and the gamma carrier waves are a blindingly fast blur. In this view, the limbic patterns emerge from the self-organizing dynamics within the space–time loop, because the critical instabilities that initiate the trajectories are located in this core of the limbic system. The patterns are then modulated by the feedback from the larger loops in which the space–time loop is embedded. These loops express the principle that transmissions between cortices are invitations to cooperate, rather than commands to perform. I therefore believe that the self-organizing evolution of AM patterns through chaotic instabilities paces the flow of intentional action. This is the main work of organizing the self. Tani used a dynamical-systems perspective to develop his view that the self emerges and exists only during the chaotic state transitions, when the deterministic machinery of linear causality (Chapter 6) is momentarily in abeyance, while a link in the externally inferred chain of cause and effect is being broken.

Although most limbic outflow goes to the sensory systems, a small fraction goes directly to two main motor systems: the amygdala (Figure 16), which directs the musculoskeletal system, and the hypothalamus, which controls the heart, lungs, skin and endocrine glands to support our muscular exertions and emotional expressions. The amygdala is known to be involved in emotional behaviour. The neuropsychologists Heinrich Klüver and Paul Bucy showed sixty years ago that removing the amygdala tamed violent monkeys and altered their feeding and sexual behaviours. Their findings led the neurosurgeons Vernon Mark, Frank Ervin and Hrdeki Narabayashi to remove the amygdala in humans to reduce violence in adults and hyperactivity in children. The outcome was that all emotional behaviours were reduced, with the patients acting like zombies. They also inserted electrodes to stimulate the amygdala of human volunteers and asked them what they felt. The replies included vague descriptions of depression, mild elation and anxiety, but, as in other similar neurosurgical studies, the results were inconclusive. This is partly because the stimuli were so different from anything the patients had experienced before that they were unable to comprehend them, and partly because neurosurgeons tend to suggest to their patients what they might expect to feel. It is impossible to impose strict psychometric controls in the operating room, and when the patients are conscious under local anaesthesia and are totally dependent on the surgeons for their lives, they intend to please them.

Recent non-invasive imaging studies have shown that the amygdala is active during the emotion of fear. It is actually involved in the expression and experience of all emotions, but it is much more difficult to elicit love, anger, jealousy, contempt or pity in subjects who are immobilized in the machinery required for functional brain imaging. Sex is problematic, because subjects must not move during imaging, so researchers or technicians would have to masturbate the research subjects in public, something grant review boards and editors of scientific journals do not support.

What is the role of the motor cortices in the frontal lobes? The limbic output goes directly by axons to the frontal lobes, and indirectly from the amygdala and hypothalamus into other parts of the basal ganglia, including the thalamus. By these routes, limbic participation is broadly established in the frontal lobes, which are motor in two senses. In the narrow sense, the motor cortices (Figure 16) control the position of the limbs, head and eyes to optimize the sensory inflow in accordance with the goal-directed actions initiated in the limbic system. But the primary motor cortices do not initiate the actions.

In the broad sense, the frontal lobe elaborates the predictions of future states and possible outcomes towards which the limbic system directs intentional action. In simple animals, there is little or no frontal cortex, and their intentional action is correspondingly impoverished. Even in cats, dogs and large-brained animals, such as elephants and whales, the frontal lobe comprises only a small fraction of each hemisphere. These animals are short-sighted and have brief attention spans. The great apes presage the emergence of the dominance of the frontal lobes in humans. In the past half-million years, the human forebrain has grown faster than any other organ in any other species in Earth's history. The dorsal and lateral areas of the frontal lobe are concerned with cognitive functions, such as logic and reasoning in prediction, and the medial and ventral areas are concerned with social skills and the capacity for interpersonal empathy. We can summarize these contributions as foresight and insight. The frontal lobes are crucial for social learning, practice, rehearsal and play in forming the detailed structure of experience that makes unique individuals. Their large, strongly interconnected populations of neurons have the capacity for self-organizing non-linear dynamics, like those of the primary sensory and limbic modules. They are active participants in shaping the complex behaviours in which humans excel, far beyond the capacities of even our closest relatives among the great apes. But to understand how they work in tandem with the thalamus, we need to explain their limbic and brainstem controls during normal behaviour.

An essential part of the self-regulatory functions of the limbic system, in addition to its use of the motor systems, is provided by neurons that secrete brain chemicals called neuromodulators. These neurons are found in a collection of chemically specialized nuclei embedded as pairs in the core of the brainstem of all vertebrates, from the simplest to the most complex (ourselves). Whereas neurotransmitters immediately excite or inhibit neurons, the neuromodulators enhance or diminish the effectiveness of the synapses, typically without having immediate excitatory or inhibitory actions of their own, and they typically bring about long-lasting changes in synaptic gains (Chapter 3). The neuromodulatory neurons receive input from many parts of the brain, but most important is their limbic input during the construction and control of intentional action. Their output axons typically branch widely and infiltrate the neuropil without making terminal synapses. They secrete their chemicals to permeate throughout the neuropil of both cerebral hemispheres, making their actions global, not local like the neurotransmitters. This functional architecture is a major determinant of the unity of intentionality, because the entire forebrain is simultaneously affected by the action of each pair of nuclei.

There are at least a dozen important neuromodulators with differing chemical structures. The types of modulation include: generalized arousal by histamine; sedation and the induction of sleep by serotonin; regulation of affect and movement by dopamine; modulation of circadian rhythms by melatonin; introduction of value by the reward hormone, CCK; relief of pain by the endorphins; release of aggressive behaviour by vasopressin; initiation of maternal behaviour by oxytocin; and facilitation of changes in synaptic gains with imprinting and learning by acetylcholine and noradrenaline (also known as norepinephrine), which is crucial for the updating stage of intentionality. These changes are cumulative, so they meet the requirement for continuing additions to the personal history constituting the evolving 'wholeness' of intentionality. When a new fact, skill or insight is learned, the widespread synaptic changes knit the modification into the entire loop, and into the entire structure of meaning that is embedded in the neuropil. Neuromodulators combine their actions to achieve states in people and animals that we describe in terms of mood, disposition, affect, attitude and temperament. It is not clear how they combine to do this, or how different proportions of the modulators are related to distinctive emotional states (Chapter 6), but we know that the neuromodulators are essential for intentional action, including emotion, and for the construction of meaning, including remembering.

The requests for cooperation sent from the limbic system to the motor systems are accompanied by transmissions of action potentials to the primary sensory cortices (Figure 18) in efference copies and corollary discharges. They are highly significant in perception, because they provide the basis on which the consequences of impending motor actions are predicted for the expected stimuli to each of the sensory ports (Chapter 2). The preafference precedes feedback by proprioception and interoception loops from the sensory receptors in the muscles and joints to the spinal cord, cerebellum, thalamus and somatosensory cortex. The corollary discharges convey information about what is to be sought by looking, listening and sniffing, and the returning afferent discharges convey the current state of the search. When an expected stimulus is present, we experience it. When it is not, we imagine it.

Preafference provides an order parameter that shapes the attractor landscapes, making it easier to capture expected or desired stimuli by enlarging or deepening the basins of their attractors. My view is that the corollary discharges do this by a macroscopic bias that tilts the sensory attractor landscapes, facilitating entry into relevant basins and their attractors. The same limbic message is sent to all the sensory cortices, so that the choice of a goal orients the senses in the same context, whether it is to find food, safety or the feeling of power and comprehension that occurs when dopamine receptors are acti-

Dynamic Architecture of the Limbic System

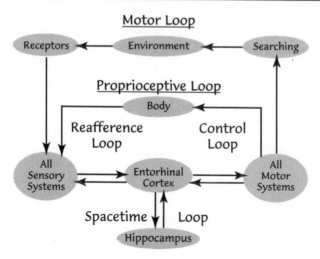

Figure 18 This diagram of the functioning brain maps the multiple feedback loops that support the intentional arc. Neural activity inside the brain flows in two directions. Forward flow from the sensory systems to the entorhinal cortex and on to the motor systems is by spatial AM patterns of action potentials at the microscopic level, which is how transmitting cortices drive the neurons in their targets. Feedback flow from the motor systems to the entorhinal cortex by control loops, and from the entorhinal cortex to the sensory systems inside the brain, is by spatial AM patterns of action potentials at the macroscopic level. This feedback constrains and modulates the microscopic activity in the forwardly transmitting populations. The macroscopic feedback messages are order parameters that bias the attractor landscapes of the sensory cortices in preafference. Forward flow supports motor output and provides the content of percepts, whereas feedback flow supports integrative processes in learning that lead to awareness and explicit memories. They enable the formation of a global AM pattern that reflects the integration of the activity of an entire hemisphere. Such global integration is the tenth building block of the dynamics of intentionality.

vated. The organism has some idea, whether correct or mistaken, of what it is looking for. The scent of prey combined with the touch of wind on the skin instantly causes the ears to listen and the eyes to look for waving grass. Preafference provides the multimodal perceptual processes of expectation and attention. Without this preconfiguration, there could be neither search nor perception. Without sensory recursion, there would be no intentional action. Without emotion, there would be no remembering.

It is generally accepted that even the simplest brains have a large number of parts, and that the parts are semi-autonomous. This means that the parts sustain and regulate their own local activity largely independently of what is going on in other parts of the brain, through the negative feedback processes of homeostasis. But they are not completely autonomous, because they do receive input from other parts and transmit their own patterns of action potentials, so they take part in the large-scale activity of the brain in which they are embedded. The spatial AM patterns in the EEGs recorded from the primary sensory areas are manifestations of their local semi-autonomous activity. Such local domains have been called 'patches' by William Calvin and 'bubbles' by John Taylor. In cortex, they are about as large as a fingernail, include millions of neurons, and flash on and off at rates of five to twenty times a second. Most researchers who do brain imaging agree that the perceptions and emotions we experience and the behaviours we observe in ourselves and others are based in the brain-wide organization of neurons in these patches. While most neurobiologists believe that behaviours and experiences are produced by either a small fraction of neurons in each patch cooperating, or by a small number of patches. So I propose that every neuron and every patch participates in every experience and behaviour, even if its contribution is to silence its pulse train or stay dark in a brain image. What is important is the small fraction of semi-autonomous activity in every part that is coordinated, not the small fraction of neurons or patches that is more active than the average.

According to several theories about brain function, a global cooperative process underlies the unity of perception and action. Neuropsychologist Karl Pribram based his interpretation on long-term studies of the effects of surgical brain lesions on the behaviour of monkeys trained to perform complex cognitive tasks. Clinical neurologist Antonio Damasio based his interpretation on his broad knowledge of the distortions of human behaviour induced by mental and neurological diseases. Most psychophysiologists agree that, whatever form it takes, wide-spread coordination must occur. Jack Pettigrew reports this from studies of binocular rivalry. When subjects are asked to look at two different images simultaneously, one in each eye, they report seeing one or the other, but not both, with the perceived images alternating sporadically. Earlier researchers concluded that the thalamus was selecting which visual cortex to activate, but Pettigrew has shown that the entire hemisphere on each side is involved globally with each alternation, as though the left and right hemispheres transfer the work of perception from one to the other like two relay runners passing a baton. Bernard Baars postulates a 'global workspace' on the basis of his analysis of the neuropsychological literature. Neurophysicist Paul Nunez proposes that the global coordination is imposed by resonant modes that depend on the boundary conditions imposed by the skull, and has described relations between intrinsic brain frequencies and brain size that support his view. Biologist Stuart Hameroff and mathematician Roger Penrose started from the premise that neurons cooperate globally. They have suggested that quantum coherence of the water bound into the internal structure of neurons is responsible, although physicists think that brains are too large and too warm to support that form of superconductivity.

I believe that hemisphere-wide cooperation is mediated by patches that interact through AM pattern transmission by axons to create a global AM pattern at a yet higher hierarchical level of activity. The patches constrain each other by sharing their local AM patterns and partially merge into a coordinated oscillation. Just as the neurons in each patch retain a high degree of autonomy, the patches within the global pattern retain substantial individual order. And just as it is difficult to detect the mesoscopic AM patterns by observing just a few neurons at a time, so the global pattern cannot be seen by measuring the output of one or a few patches. We must deduce it from measurements of global brain images.

These images have come within our reach in the past decade by applying massive computer processing to the raw materials of observation. One source is the use of computer graphics to display patterns of regional blood flow detected by functional magnetic resonance imaging (fMRI), exemplified by the work of Per Roland. Most displays are made by subtracting two successive brain images of each subject, one of which was taken while the subject performed a cognitive task, such as doing mental arithmetic. The differences between the images show as bright spots on a picture of the brain that suggest localization of the function to one or a few patches. But these differences are deceptive. The true picture is that the global activity of the brain has regions of high and low activity in every task, and that changes between tasks occur in the same way that AM patterns change, with new locations of high and low levels of activity. Moreover, fMRI displays are static, virtually anatomical, and cannot reveal the rapid sequences of state transitions that occur as global AM patterns evolve.

Better sources of images are the electrical and magnetic fields of potential measured by the electroencephalogram (EEG) and the magnetoencephalogram (MEG), which have the required degrees of spatial and temporal resolution. There are many examples of these techniques being used successfully, including the demonstration by Dietrich Lehmann of global spatial patterns of alpha waves with state transitions five times each second, on average, in the scalp EEGs of human volunteers. And Urs Ribary and Rodolfo Llinás found global gamma waves in the MEGs in awake humans. Catherine Tallon-Baudry, Mathias Müller, Francisco Varela and their colleagues have shown that patterns of gamma activity in scalp recordings are closely related to visual attention and cognition. Their findings show that the distance from the cortex to the recording sites outside the head, imposed by the scalp and skull, actually improves access by observers to the spatially coherent activity of global AM patterns, because the spatial summation that blurs the local activity lets us see the shared components of the global activity. Everyone knows that if you get too close to a newsprint picture, you see only meaningless dots.

Examples from animal research include large-scale patterns

uniting the visual and motor cortices shown in dogs by Vera Dumenko, in monkeys by Steve Bressler and Richard Nakamura, and in cats, rats and rabbits by myself and my students, Leslie Kay, John Barrie, Paul German and others. Many neurobiologists have found widespread coordination in the timing of action potentials in the neocortex, which must exist because the local AM patterns are carried by pulses. Moshe Abeles and his colleagues record from widely separated neurons in the neocortex of monkeys that perform skilled tasks for which they are specially trained, and find 'synfire chains' of precisely timed pulses. Wolf Singer and his colleagues find synchronization of the firing of feature-detector neurons in the visual system, which enables the binding of information into representations of objects. So, many researchers, using various techniques, have found evidence for global AM patterns. Now we need to know what properties these global patterns have, how they form, and what role they play in the genesis of intentional behaviour.

The formation of global AM patterns indicates that the sensorimotor and limbic areas of each hemisphere can rapidly enter into a cooperative state, which persists for perhaps a tenth of a second before dissolving to make way for the next state. This cooperation does not develop by entrainment of coupled oscillators into synchronous oscillation, as resonance is much too slow and the linear correlations between the waveforms from the different locations stay well above chance levels and do not fluctuate significantly. But it is not the level of correlation that changes with perception and action, but the global AM pattern, as the cooperation carries the entire hemisphere from one global chaotic attractor to the next. The genesis of macroscopic chaos by interacting brain parts does not require that they oscillate with identical waveforms having linear correlations.

At the moment we have no clear measure of the degree of correlation that patches must reach to form a global order parameter that can successfully constrain those patches and bring the billions of neurons that make up each human cerebral hemisphere into global order within a few thousandths of a second. Although no cortical neuron is more than a few synapses from any other, so brains can form what Duncan Watts and Steven Strogatz call 'small worlds', the transmission distances over which cooperation is established are thousands of times greater than the diameters of spread of the axons and dendrites of all but a few neurons. The forebrains of simpler vertebrates, such as the salamander, are smaller than the human olfactory bulb. In such small forebrains we can easily see how globally coherent oscillatory states form. But the brains of small mammals, such as rabbits and cats, are enormous by comparison, and the time needed to send pulses between cortical modules is too great to allow continuous widespread synchronization of pulse trains, although many instances are observed. The brains of humans, elephants and whales boggle the imagination.

The mammalian neocortex, which supports the cooperation we detect in global AM patterns, has two properties that help to explain the rapid formation of unified global states. The first property is the presence of large projection neurons in the deeper layers. Neocortex is commonly described anatomically as having six layers (Figure 3) of cell bodies, whereas the archicortex (hippocampus) and the palaeocortex (the bulb and olfactory cortex) are said to have three layers. Functionally, the older forms of cortex are actually a single layer of projection neurons and interneurons, with input axons coming into the superficial side and output axons leaving in the deep side. The six cell layers in the neocortex have two such functional sheets. The input and output axons enter and leave in the deep side. The outer functional sheet, containing cell layers I to III, is similar in many respects to the palaeocortex. The inner functional sheet, containing layers IV to VI, has fewer projection neurons that are many times larger than those of the outer sheet. The long apical dendrites (Figure 4) penetrate all six layers, and the basal dendrites radiate widely in all directions in the sheet. These large neurons integrate the cortical activity over much larger cortical areas than do the superficial cells, their axons project much farther, and their action potentials travel at much higher conduction velocities. These large, deep-lying cells provide the anatomical and functional bases for long-range interactions between patches, which are the macroscopic local neighbourhoods of the neocortex. They are like satellite links between cities that all have local telephone networks.

The other important property of the neocortex is that it is a continuous sheet of neuropil covering each hemisphere. There are obvious architectural differences in the neuropil between the many local areas of neocortex, which are labelled in various schemes, the most widely used being that of Korbinian Brodmann. But these different areas merge into each other without any loss in the densities of axonal and dendritic branches or their synaptic connections. The neocortex is not united in this way with the palaeocortex, the archicortex (hippocampus), or the opposite cerebral hemisphere, which are connected by axonal tracts. This anatomical characteristic supports the formation of global AM patterns in the neocortex of small mammals. How it suffices in the brains of humans is still a matter for conjecture, as we have not yet made the necessary measurements of the electrical and magnetic fields of pulse and wave potentials from various cortical sites throughout each hemisphere.

In conclusion, I propose that global interaction occurs at the highest of the three hierarchical levels of brain activity. The full meaning of a stimulus for the organism emerges from the cortical neuropil only at the global level. Meaning depends on the entire history of an animal, which is embedded in the neuropil by synaptic modifications during learning. The meaning is shaped by the present context, which is provided by the senses of the body and the world under limbic control, and it includes the states of emotion and affect that are implemented by the neuro-modulatory nuclei of the brainstem, also under limbic control, in preparation for the execution of intended actions, particularly social interactions that require non-verbal signalling. The same global states that embody the meaning provide the AM patterns that make choices between available options and that guide the motor systems into sequential movements of intentional behaviour. In Chapter 6 we shall consider the role of this global AM pattern in the formation of meaning, particularly in relation to awareness and consciousness.

Awareness, consciousness, and causality

The biology of meaning includes the entire brain and body, with the history built by experience into bones, muscles, endocrine glands and neural connections. A meaningful state is an activity pattern of the nervous system and body that has a particular focus in the state space of the organism, not in the physical space of the brain. As meaning changes, the focus changes, forming a trajectory that jumps, bobs and weaves like the course of a firefly on a summer night. The elements of each dynamic state consist of the pulses and waves in the brain, the contractions of the muscles, the joint angles of the skeletal system, and the secretions of cells in the autonomic and neuroendocrine systems. Meanings emerge from the whole of the synaptic connections among the neurons of the neuropil, the sensitivities of their trigger zones, determined by the neuromodulators, and to lesser extents the growth, form and adaptations of the rest of the body. The skills of athletes, dancers and musicians live not only in their synapses, but also in their limbs, fingers and torsos. Neurobiologists who study the molecular basis of learning in synapses tend to overlook the fact that enlarged muscles and honed immune systems have also learned to do their jobs.

The strengths of connections between the neurons and the properties of the body are continually shaped by learning and exercise throughout a lifetime. Each of us is born with genetic and cytoplasmic endowments that establish some general limits to the directions and extents of growth in striving for the wholeness of intentionality. A state of meaning then knits together the brain and body in brief time intervals, which, in the language of neurodynamics, form short segments of an itinerant trajectory through the state space of the organism. This state space includes the range of possible actions begun at any moment by the personal history and condition of the organism, its wholeness. Each segment has a location in state space and a preferred direction given by the trajectory. To define that location, we must determine the state through measurements of brain and behaviour. We can do this by choosing successive pairs of state variables, such as the firing rate of motor neurons and the speed of running, or the firing rate of sensory neurons and the brightness of a light. As we build increasingly complex arrays of measurements, the relevance of each variable to all the others reflects the unity of the intentional actions that establish meaning. The trajectory of transitions through brain states in an organism embodies the steps towards an end state or goal, that is already part of the meaning. So meaning reflects three properties of intentional behaviour: wholeness, unity and intent.

Meaning is also a state of mind that we all experience through observations of our own actions and those of others. Awareness is an experience, which in neurodynamic terms is a transient state. Consciousness is the process by which sequences of hemisphere-wide states of awareness form a trajectory of meaning. Our experiences of trajectories encompass sequences ranging from the strict and orderly flow of logical deduction, through habit or strong concentration, to the turbulence of streams of consciousness in idle play and dreams. We know this through our own streams of consciousness, and through perceiving the representations of others' experiences and thoughts in drama, poetry, art, films, novels, journals, scientific texts, and the social exchanges of daily life. Unlike the activities of brains and bodies, which we can measure and express in numbers, experiences cannot be represented in tables and graphs. But we can describe them in words and works of art. The systematic study of experiences is known as phenomenology.

We can also describe the dynamics of brains and bodies in words instead of numbers, as I have done in the preceding chapters. The task of understanding the relations between experiences and brain activities then consists in finding correspondences between two verbal constructs: phenomenology and neuroscience. This is commonly called the mind–body problem, but that formulation is a pseudo-problem. Posing a causal connection between an intellect and a material substance results in a category error. We usually think of problems as having solutions, but a pseudo-problem has none, and if it did, the solution would be different for everyone because the neurodynamics and meanings are unique in each brain. But the local correspondences between brain activities and experiences are important and can be described, and here we are concerned with their descriptions.

We shall now have a look at some of the relations between the neural and mental dynamics of awareness. There is no need to prove that a biological connection exists, because most of us have used chemicals and drugs, in substances such as wine, tea or tobacco, to modify, enhance or suppress states of awareness in medicinal, religious or recreational contexts. So what is this connection? How do states of awareness change the activities of neurons? How can neural activity cause awareness, which include states of pain or pleasure? These are questions of cause and effect. Causality is implicit and unavoidable in the underlying question with which I began: who or what controls your brain? These questions can be answered with words serving as representations, but only by exploring the conceptual framework of causality in which they are asked. The key to capturing causality lies in understanding how we experience the intentionality by which meaning is created.

We do not usually think of intentionality as something that can be experienced, because analytic philosophers, who currently claim exclusive possession of the word, use it to mean something very abstract. Phenomenology was introduced and

developed by European philosophers in the first half of the twentieth century as a systematic attempt to escape from the tradition
of introspection. In this tradition, as it was devised by Immanuel
Kant, the mind consists of innate ideas derived by pure reason,
and the world of objects and events exists independently of
observers. In this Kantian view the task of philosophers is to
reason from their raw sense data and thereby shape our ideas
about the world. We are subjects thinking about objects.

Early phenomenologists, such as Franz Brentano and Edmund
Husserl, accepted the idea from Kant that the contents of the
mind have the form of representations of the world, but they
objected to the premise that the mind has innate ideas, because
there is too much cultural variation in the world. They decided
that ideas must come from experience, so they tried to describe
accurately, and without cultural or personal biases, the relations
between the ideas in their minds and the things in the world
that they represent. Brentano reintroduced Thomas Aquinas'
concept of intentionality to designate these relations, in which
a thought or a belief or an idea is 'about' the world. He did this
to distinguish between people, who know what they are doing,
and logical machines, that do not. In this view, which is today the
most common among Anglo-American analytic philosophers,
representations are states of mind, and we are conscious of them,
so consciousness precedes intentionality. Consciousness is also
the property that cognitivists would like to build into intelligent
machines, which is why they are so concerned with what they
call the mystery of consciousness. Some scientists, such as
Whitehead and Penrose, go further by proposing that consciousness is an essential property of all matter along with energy
and mass, and that brains have advanced forms of consciousness
simply because their atoms and quantum particles are organized
in interesting ways. But some philosophers dismiss this view as
'panexperientialism' or 'panpsychism', an early and widespread
belief in animism, that objects are inhabited by spirits.

Phenomenology flourished in a bizarre direction in the middle
of the twentieth century through the popularization by Aldous
Huxley and Tim Leary of hallucinogens, such as LSD, magic

mushrooms, and related drugs, which were alleged to help 'open the doors of perception' and allow people to get as close as possible to the raw sense data of experience. The preprocessing that is normally done by the educated perceptual systems could be short-circuited so, with pharmacological assistance, anybody willing to take the trip could unload a lot of cultural baggage and see the world 'as it really is, infinite', (as William Blake put it in *The Marriage of Heaven and Hell*). They saw amazing colours in pulsing spirals and experienced some unusual perceptual distortions and out-of-body phenomena already known to clinical neurologists, and they contributed to the neuropharmacology of altered brain states. But mainstream phenomenologists sought bigger game.

Martin Heidegger, one of Husserl's students, broke from Kant's position by proposing that human ideas come from the everyday actions and concerns that make up human existence in time. He located the basis for human intelligence within the ordered structures of society in which people find themselves as they emerge into consciousness. He referred to their status in these structures as their 'throwness'. These structures are not the independent mental forms proposed by Plato, Descartes and Kant, nor are they representations, but come into being through the actions people take to cope with their surroundings. In other words, intentionality precedes consciousness, and the dichotomy between subject and object disappears. Action precedes perception. As Napoleon remarked, when asked how he succeeded in battle: 'On s'engage, y puis on vois', ('You jump in and then see what to do').

A similar approach was taken by Jean Piaget in his analyses of psychomotor development. In the somatomotor phase during their first two years, children learn about the world using their bodies to explore it by 'stretching forth'. Heidegger's follower Merleau-Ponty investigated the biological foundation for social experience by using descriptions from the neurologists Goldstein and Gelb of the syndromes they observed in patients with brain damage incurred during the First World War. Their clinical data provided him with a window into the normal unity of human

skills from the ways in which that unity breaks down in patients
with injured brains. Repeatedly, the clinicians showed that local-
ized brain damage in any of a variety of brain regions caused
patients to exhibit generalized impairment across a wide variety
of behaviours. An example of such an informative dysfunction
was the loss by a patient of the ability to point to an object,
which is a social action intended to inform someone else, while
retaining the ability to grasp it, which is the utilitarian assimilation by the body of some part of the world. From this evidence,
Merleau-Ponty hypothesized that perception is a focus in the
structure of learned behaviour, which becomes explicit as an
organized multisensory perception when the organism applies its
skills by acting into the world. He concluded that philosophical
biases inherent in 'empiricism' and 'intellectualism' – the precursors of materialism and cognitivism – had prevented his pre-
decessors from recognizing the ways that human mental
activities shape themselves by adapting bodily movements
towards biological goals in everyday tasks.

When asked at the end of a long and exhausting conference to
sum up the principle of his view, Merleau-Ponty replied: 'To
perceive is to render oneself present to something through the
body.' This sentence conveyed the main elements of what he
was talking about. He elaborated: 'All the while the thing keeps
its place within the horizon of the world, and the structuring
consists of putting each detail in the perceptual horizons which
belong to it.' This description, whether he intended it to or not,
clearly conforms to Aquinas' process of assimilation, by which
the brain learns about an object by making itself similar in
selected aspects to the object through organization of the body
and neurons throughout the brain. He appears to make a distinction between the horizon of the world outside and the
horizon of perception within. In terms of dynamics, a person can
act onto and change an object, but that object does not cross its
own horizon into the brain and imprint its features through the
inner horizon of the sensory cortices, in the sense that one can
move towards a horizon but can never reach it. If my interpretation is correct, he grasped the concept of the uni-

directionality and the solipsistic isolation that it portends, because the forms in matter, according to Aquinas, cannot be grasped directly. All that we can know comes through the imagination, which allows us to generalize and abstract to create the internal structures with which we act and understand.

The act of perception transcends the two horizons through assimilation. Our perception of an object has already been conceived before the sensory input, by the action taken to obtain the input. The structuring is done by repeated cycles of action and perception that Merleau-Ponty calls the intentional arc, which constitutes the effort to achieve maximum grip. His 'putting each detail' within the perceptual horizon essentially means positioning the sensory receptors through efference and focusing the sensory cortices through preafference, which is to pay attention in order to achieve optimal assimilation of the self to an object. The self adapts to that object and learns about it by shaping the body, and also by reshaping or repositioning the object. A familiar example is manipulating a new tool with our fingers, squeezing it, inspecting its facets visually, listening to the sound it makes when it is tapped, and then applying it to other objects, as we conceive and configure them.

Merleau-Ponty concludes that we are moved to action by a disequilibrium between the self and the world. In dynamic terms, the disequilibrium is an endogenous instability that puts the brain onto an itinerant trajectory, that is, a pathway through a chain of preferred states, which are learned basins of attraction. The penultimate result is not an equilibrium in the chemical sense, which is a dead state, but a descent for a time into the basin of an attractor, giving an awareness of closure.

There is something implicit in phenomenology that I want to make explicit. The aim of phenomenology is to describe sensory experiences without metaphysical preconceptions. These sensory experiences must come into awareness before the phenomenologists can abstract, examine and represent them in words and pictures as a part of science. Essentially, it is simply impossible to talk about phenomenology, which is the study, reflection upon and knowledge about phenomena, without invoking awareness, because that is the medium through which we experience these constructions and represent them in words. Phenomenologists are clearly conscious and aware as an active part of their own structuring process of assimilation. But Merleau-Ponty did not include awareness as a requirement for structuring in the daily activities defining intelligence. He referred only occasionally to consciousness, and even less often to awareness. In at least one passage, he treated consciousness as an epiphenomenon that was unsuitable for scientific study, in contrast with the concreteness of the intentional arc. But science and scientists cannot function without talk and awareness, so we are well advised not to dismiss awareness or sweep it under the phenomenological rug.

Neurodynamicists think in terms of space and time, so we ask whether awareness is present throughout the intentional arc, or whether it arises in one segment of the arc (Figures 17 and 18), and if so, which one? How much time is required for one passage around the intentional arc, and how long after the onset of an action or a stimulus does a volunteer report becoming aware of it? Everyone agrees that perception takes time. Minimal estimates of the time between warning stimuli and learned responses, given by measuring the reaction times of humans and animals, range from a quarter to three quarters of a second. These are longer than the reaction times between painful or rewarding stimuli and responses that require no learning, which are less than a tenth of a second. Only a small fraction of the delay in responding to learned stimuli is taken up by delays in axonal conduction between receptors and the brain, between the brain parts, and from the brain to the muscles. Materialists and cognitivists say that most of the interval is required for information processing, which includes binding features into higher-order images, and for retrieving and matching stored representations by cross-correlation with the present input. Pragmatists think that the interval is required for the brain parts to seek appropriate basins of attraction, and for the attractors to construct AM patterns in an itinerant trajectory that integrates the different parts of the forebrain.

Clearly, awareness of a stimulus is not simultaneous with the onset of the stimulus, nor does it precede the genesis of an action. Experiments to measure the time to awareness were conducted by neurophysiologist Benjamin Libet in collaboration with neurosurgeons. Libet took advantage of the fact that there are two somatosensory pathways from the spinal cord to the cortex. The ascending axons in the lemniscal pathway are fast and unbranched, and almost instantly report to the cortex exactly where and when a stimulus hits the skin. In contrast, the axons in the spinothalamic pathway are slow and branch extensively through relays into the limbic system and through the thalamic reticular formation to all parts of the forebrain. These axons initiate the process that leads to perceiving the stimulus half a second later.

To diagnose and treat intractable epilepsy, the neurosurgeons placed electrodes in the brains of patients, who volunteered to stay awake while their brains were exposed under local anaesthesia so they could report their perceptions of direct electrical stimulation of their sensory cortices. In some trials, the surgeons stimulated a nerve in the left hand of patients, which evoked an electrical response in the right sensory cortex almost instantly by the fast pathway. The patients reported feeling the stimulus half a second later. In other trials, the surgeons electrically stimulated the exposed left sensory cortex, which bypassed the fast pathway from the right hand but caused an immediate sensory cortical response. Once again, about a half second elapsed before the patients reported perceiving the stimulus, despite the immediate evoked potential.

Two outcomes of Libet's experiment are especially significant. First, the stimulus given to the left hand could be felt no matter how brief it was, but the stimulus given directly to the left cortex had to be a pulse train that lasted at least a quarter to a half a second to achieve what Libet called 'neuronal adequacy' for awareness. Briefer durations required higher stimulus intensities. Second, the awareness of the direct electrical stimulus to the left cortex was assigned by the patients to the end of the pulse train, the time for 'neuronal adequacy', but awareness of the stimulus given to the left hand, activating the lemniscal pathway, was 'backdated' to its time of occurrence. In fact, neurobiologists have been mystified for years about what exactly the lemniscal pathway does, and here it is. Its backdating keeps brain function concurrent with the flow of real time, despite the obligatory delay in the formation of a percept. Anyone who plays on a sports team or in an orchestra can see how important it is to keep rapid sequences of behaviour in harmony with the group, at rates of change too fast to allow perceptual frames in succession, yet requiring integration into the shared time sequences of the unfolding events.

Although Libet's experiments have been severely criticized for lack of accurate measures of inner awareness, the fact is that the process of awareness is more complex than the induced state transition in a sensory cortex and takes more time. The solipsistic isolation makes measuring the time to awareness difficult because the only way that neurobiologists can know when other people are conscious, is to ask: 'What did you feel, and when did you feel it?' The same problem makes it difficult to estimate the time at which an awareness of the intent to act emerges. Libet and others, have deduced from measurements of brain activity in human volunteers that a comparable delay exists in the awareness of intent to perform a self-paced action. In this case, a slow change in electric potential is recorded using scalp electrodes between the top of the head and the base at the earlobes. When the neurologists ask an experimental subject to press a switch briefly, at his or her own pace, now and then over the course of an hour, they find a slow increase in a 'readiness potential' that starts about a second before each self-paced movement. The potential change is so small that it can be detected only by averaging over numerous trials, but it shows that neural activity involved in the planning and organization of the movement precedes the awareness of an intention to act. The length of time between the onset of the readiness potential and awareness is comparable to the delay in the awareness of a stimulus onset. That is, when the subjects are asked to report the time of onset of their awareness of the decision to initiate pressing the switch, the timing of their responses indicates that their awareness follows the onset of the readiness potential by between a quarter and half a second. Brain activity preceding the initiation of an intentional act starts before the onset of awareness of an intent to engage in that action. The subjects also report that, after becoming aware that they are about to act, they can abort the action. This is rather like becoming aware of what you are about to say and deciding to modify it or censor it. So, whoever or whatever you are, your awareness is one of your assets and tools, not the agency that initiates action.

James came to a similar conclusion when he described waking and lying in bed in the morning, telling himself to get up. Nothing happened. He stayed in bed. He later found himself up and about but could not remember getting up. Merleau-Ponty, after his review of Goldstein and Gelb's neurological evidence, also inferred that awareness follows action rather than preceding it. He wrote: 'It is clear that no causal relationship is conceivable between the subject and his body, his world and his society.' He reasoned that consciousness lay outside the action–perception cycle. He added: 'What misleads us on this is that we often look for freedom, free will, in the voluntary deliberation which examines one motive after another and seems to opt for the weightiest or most convincing. In reality, the deliberation follows the decision and it is my secret decision which brings the motives to life.' Secret from whom? Secret even from our own awareness, so that we make decisions and then justify, rationalize and explain them afterwards with our deliberations. In his view, consciousness is not the cause of a decision, nor is it an effect, but a relation between cause and effect, which is a mental process.

He proposed that actions are not controlled by consciousness, because experience has already created an understanding of the present, from which action flows without need for reflection. Awareness is not essential for intentional coping, because many of our daily actions emerge without reflection. But doing science is not among them, and phenomenology is incomplete unless we describe it as a dynamic process emerging within neurons and populations. I therefore want to raise the question of how to understand awareness and consciousness in neurobiological terms. For that, I need three premises.

The first premise is uncontroversial: the brain is a dynamic system. Each state of awareness occupies a space–time synaptic field that has patterns of pulse and wave densities and their electrochemical components distributed through the brain. Each frame has a place in a sequence through brain state space. This sequence is the trajectory of a state variable, which expresses the synaptic residues of past acts of perception, and which leads to new acts of perception. Consciousness, then, is both a mental process experienced phenomenologically and a neural process that links and embeds this sequence of brain states, so it is not just a state variable in the brain. It is also what engineers call an operator that mediates relations among neurons. Far from being an epiphenomenon, excretion, accident or sideshow, it must play a crucial role in intentional behaviour. It is the task of neurodynamicists to define and measure what that role is.

My second premise is that awareness and consciousness exist in animals with degrees of variation in content and complexity that correspond to the varieties of structures and functions found in brains throughout the animal kingdom. In humans, consciousness takes different forms, owing to the complexity of human brains and human social activity. Yet irrespective of the contents, the fundamental state variable-operator, and the role it plays in structuring intentional behaviour, should be found in all vertebrates. The proof, obviously, cannot be sought by asking animals to describe what they experience in states of awareness, if they have any. But I believe we can infer the nature of the operation from analyses of the dynamics of animal brains, even if we cannot know directly the contents, namely, what they are thinking.

My third premise is that consciousness can be understood only in the light of a sufficient understanding of causality. Here are the usual questions. How do actions cause perceptions? How do perceptions cause awareness? How do states of awareness cause actions? To these, I want to add some more. Why do we ask them in this way? How is it that we find satisfaction in answers that give us the 'causes' of things as explanations? Is this good science, seeing that from an early age we are taught that scientists ask 'how?' and not 'why?'

Analysis of causality is a necessary step towards understanding consciousness, because the forms our answers take depend on the choice among three meanings that we assign to 'cause'. The first is to make, move or modulate, as by an agency, which corresponds to Aristotle's efficient cause, in which a person causes an accident, a germ causes a disease, and so on. This is 'why'. I refer to this meaning as linear causality. The second meaning is to explain, rationalize or blame, corresponding to Aristotle's formal cause. In common with many physicists and psychologists, I refer to this meaning as 'circular causality'. This is the context in which we use the word 'because' to denote an explanation without invoking an agency. This is 'how'. The third is to treat causality as a human trait that we assign to objects and events in the world. This was the conclusion reached by David Hume in the eighteenth century. He based his view in a philosophical doctrine called 'nominalism', holding that abstract concepts and generalizations are properties of minds, not of the world. He concluded that knowledge of causes is solely the result of constant conjunctions of events in sequences. Remarkably, the same conclusion on the same premise was reached by Aquinas four centuries earlier, that the forms in the intellect are created by the imagination and do not exist in the forms taken by matter. I have used his conclusion to explain the unidirectionality of perception, in which the forms taken by brain activity in the sensory cortices are created internally, not imposed by the forms of stimuli. In this view, causality is a quale, the feeling of necessity. It is a threshold in the degree of the certainty of prediction that we assign to an observed relation in terms of what it portends for our own future actions.

Linear causality is what we usually mean when we think about causes. When we interpret events according to this view, we assign to each event a beginning and an end. Behaviourists call the beginning a stimulus and the end a response. Cognitivists in artificial intelligence, neural networks and computational neuroscience call them a cause and an effect, and sometimes they call them the independent and dependent variables. An invariant relation must hold for us to claim that a stimulus causes a response. To show invariance, we must give the same stimulus repeatedly and find the same response. If it does not follow, then some unknown influence has intruded and obscured the underlying constancy, so we must find it and eliminate it, like an inquisitor rooting out sin. We constantly guard against spurious conjunctions of events when they are joint effects that are caused by something else, and we eliminate them by using controlled experiments. We are constantly reminded that correlation is not causation. The invariant temporal order is crucial, because an effect can never precede its cause. Some scientists call this 'time's arrow' and use it to identify causal connections.

Each effect must become a cause for another effect, so we can build linear causal chains. For example, neurobiologists investigate the chain of neural events between a stimulus and a response. They find that the delivery of a stimulus provides information that activates the molecules in the membranes of receptor cells, which by a biochemical cascade causes transmission of the information by action potentials into the spinal cord. A chain of synapses and axons relays the information to the sensory cortices. The information is processed in several steps and carried through the frontal lobes into the motor systems, where further steps cause muscle contractions and a response (Figure 16). Through repeated observation and measurement, including randomly alternating trials in which the stimulus is omitted, researchers collect input–output pairs, from which they infer the causal chain of operations.

Although this is a familiar procedure, it is problematic. Time is supposed to be continuous through a study of input–output relations, but in practice it is fractured by the investigators because they stop the clock and restart it with each new trial. In order to make the repeated observations required to establish linear causality, they must wait for each preceding response to end – and for the organism to return to its original prestimulus condition – before they give the next stimulus. But that requirement holds only approximately, because experimental subjects change to some extent with every stimulus they perceive. Typically, a causal chain is not invariant, and researchers have to explain how the chain fails. If an expected response does not follow a stimulus, the subject under study may be fatigued, satiated, bored or distracted, or there may be a breakdown somewhere in the measuring instruments. Investigators control these conditions as best they can, and then they assign a statistical probability to the outcome. They also recognize the likelihood that, in fact, many conditions must be satisfied to create any statistical relation, and so they invoke multiple causes that feed into their primary causal chain. So we have statistical causality, in which risk factors meet the need for prediction, and multiple causality when the chain sprouts branches. When all else fails, they assert that unexpected events are caused by chance. Medical people have a special word for an unexplained disease: we call it 'agnogenic', meaning that it must have a cause but we don't know what it is. This contrasts with 'iatrogenic', which means that we caused it.

Linear causality fails most dramatically in studies of the relations between microscopic neurons and the macroscopic populations in which they are embedded. Each neuron acts onto a myriad of others within one to a few synaptic links, and already the returning impact of those others alters its state before it can send another pulse. This hierarchical interaction cannot be reduced to a linear causal chain. Such interactions are not peculiar to neurons in neuropil, being common in familiar systems such as hurricanes, lasers, fires, herds of animals, crowds of people, and so forth. In each of these cases, particles making up the ensemble simultaneously create a macroscopic state and are constrained by the very state they have created. Simultaneity violates the requirement that effects must follow causes, and the distributed nonlinear feedback makes a mockery of any attempt to determine which neuron caused which others to fire or not to fire. Scientists who study nonlinear phenomena are fond of saying that a butterfly flapping its wings in the Amazon jungle can cause a hurricane to hit Florida. This is idle conjecture, a metaphor from linear causality that they use to dramatize the sensitivity of their computational models. A better description for the relation between neurons and neuron populations is provided by circular causality.

We can also invoke circular causality to explain the interactions at a higher level among patches and populations of neurons, such as between the entorhinal cortex and hippocampus, and, still higher, in the entire action–perception cycle of the intentional arc, but with a very human touch. When we represent such interactions, whether in words as I am doing now, or with equations, or with geometrical or physical models, we use the tool of a closed loop to describe activity flowing with time in one direction around the loop. Then, in order to understand the loop, we break it into its forward and feedback limbs, and use linear causality to describe the operation in each of the two limbs. In other words, we fall back on linear causality, because that is how we experience our brains at work. It is the form of explanation with which most humans are most comfortable.

For this reason, we continue to ask in what sense awareness can cause changes in the neural activity that is shaping intentional behaviour, and how it is that, after the abatement of the sensory activity, newly structured neural activity can cause new awareness. Of course, we can declare, as Merleau-Ponty did, that causality does not enter into the relations of awareness to neural activity, or, as David Hume did, that cause is merely the sense that comes from observing constant conjunction. Or we can divide the meaning of the word 'cause', and distinguish between a cause as a reason or excuse, and a cause as an agent. On the one hand, linear causal chains always postulate agents; for example, 'an asteroid hit the Earth and caused a dust cloud that blocked off the Sun, killed the plants, and starved the dinosaurs', or 'someone pulled a trigger and caused a bullet to pierce another person, which caused that person to die'. On the other hand, circular causality offers an explanation without agency, but when we try to understand neural interactions in terms of circular causality, we make feedback loops and fall back to linear causality. A way to understand this trait is to ask why humans demand causes as explanations.

So, we have seen that an intentional act arises as a self-organized state in a segment of a trajectory that has a location in state space and a direction towards a future state. The present state is an activity pattern that incorporates the motor systems, the motions of the limbs, the sense organs, and the perceptual brain modules. The action does not need to be accompanied by awareness, but if it is, we experience the intent to act through pre-afference of the expected consequences of the act. Then we experience the act through its proprioceptive and exteroceptive consequences. Each action is in essence an experiment by which we test a hypothesis: 'if I do this, then I expect that to occur'. So we experience the intent to act as a 'cause', and we become aware of the consequences of the act as an 'effect'. We experience our action, or, more precisely, our intention to act, as causing the sensory input, or, more precisely, the constructions that follow the sensory input. According to developmental psychologists such as Piaget, we learn this relation in the sensorimotor phase early in life, well before we acquire the language and logic to describe and question it.

The attribution of causal agency by humans to other humans is essential for social organization and control, because it is the basis for assigning responsibility, with credit and reward or blame and punishment, individually and collectively. Most of us act in the belief that our actions cause the changes in the world we intend, and that someone or something else causes the changes we do not intend. Most of us regard animals and inanimate objects as having the causal power to produce effects. By extrapolation, the entire universe appears as a gigantic causal engine, having its first cause in the Big Bang, or in the Prime Mover, depending on your system of beliefs.

This alternative view is that causality has its origin in the neural mechanisms of intentionality, through which all knowledge comes, rather than existing in the world outside ourselves. Our attribution of causes to objects resembles animism. Animistic thinkers posit spirits in inanimate objects as agencies that make things happen in the world. This practice originates far too deeply in the prelingual experience of every one of us to be regarded lightly or comfortably disposed of because, without this logical crutch, we might not understand anything at all. We tend to be paralysed when we lose belief in the efficacy of our own actions, especially when we compound the loss by seeing ourselves as corks bobbing on a stormy sea or by surrendering to Spinoza's view that we like are stones rolling downhill. It takes a heroic effort to continue to live and work under such resignation to a fully deterministic world view. Most people are simply not resigned.

The question here is how to avoid assigning linear causality and agency to neurons and neural populations. There are precedents for breaking away from linear thinking, and into relational thinking, which might serve as models. An example is the animistic view of the Sun being dragged across the sky by an agent of the gods. Scientists came to realize that, in fact, we are observing the Sun from a place on a rotating sphere, and that we experience a time-varying geometric relation between the rotation of the Earth and this object far from us. This is not a causal relation. What scientists needed and used in achieving this insight was an enlarged conceptual framework that is expressed in the acausal language of differential equations and tensor calculus, and that shifted the ancient anthropocentric viewpoint from a focus in the Earth to a new and distributed network in the sky. The Solar System is not pulled together by the agency of gravity; it is structured by curved space–time.

Neurodynamics offers just such a new and enlarged conceptual framework, in which interrelations among parts creating wholes can be described without a need for causal agents. An elementary example is the self organization of a neural population by its component neurons. The neuropil in each area of cortex contains millions of neurons interacting by synaptic transmission. The density of action is low, diffuse and widespread. Under the impact of sensory stimulation, by the release from other parts of the brain of neuromodulatory chemicals, and by the background process of growth and maturation, all the neurons come together and form a macroscopic pattern of activity. This pattern simultaneously constrains the activities of the neurons that support it. The microscopic activity flows in one direction, upwards in the hierarchy, and simultaneously the macroscopic activity flows in the other direction, downwards. With the arrival of a new stimulus, or under the impact of a new condition, an entire hemisphere can be destabilized, so it jumps into a new state, and then into another, and another, then trading back and forth between the hemispheres in a sequence forming a trajectory. There is no meaning to the question of how individual neurons cause global state transitions, any more than it is meaningful to ask how some air and water molecules or a butterfly can cause a hurricane, or how a few rocks can cause an undersea earthquake and a tsunami.

Ever since Ludwig Boltzmann created statistical mechanics by joining the theory of molecules with classical thermodynamics in the nineteenth century, the acausal, hierarchical way of thinking about matter has become so familiar to physicists that it is difficult to see why it is not better understood and used by neurobiologists working with neurons. One reason (or cause) is that we can assume that all molecules of the same substance are alike, but we know that no two neurons are identical. Another reason is that linear causality works well in the reductionist direction, in which the links in causal chains are taken progressively from organs to the levels of cells, organelles, molecules, atoms and down to quantum potentia. But causal chains cannot be built in the same way in the upward direction. A reductionist is like a scientist who understands how water percolates into the ground, but cannot understand how trees can suck it up and breathe it out to fall again as rain, and who puts circular causality in the same logical category as circular reasoning. But the facts we gain continue to baffle us until we assemble them in new paradigms. All the great advances in modern science, such as the Copernican theory of the solar system, the periodic table of the elements, Rudolph Virchow's cellular doctrine of pathology, and theories of gravity, evolution, relativity and quantum mechanics, are relational systems of thought. Adding causality to them can do mischief, like for instance, the postulates of ether to carry gravity, of hidden variables to quantum theory, and of natural selection as the agency of evolution, which Darwin modelled on the artificial selection by animal breeders, and which caused the havoc of social Darwinism. Causality is in the minds of humans, not in the malevolence of nature.

How can a human or other animal be a causal agent? The answer comes from brain dynamics. The primary sensory cortices are all components of a larger network, together with the various parts of the limbic system. Each of these components is liable to destabilization at any time, because of the interaction of populations by axonal feedback connections. Perception can, and often does, follow the impact of sensory bombardment, but that which is perceived has already been prepared for in two ways. The first way is by the residue of past experience, the synaptic modifications that shape the connections in the neuropil of each sensory cortex to form nerve-cell assemblies. Each assembly opens the door to a preferred spatial pattern that is constructed by the learned attractor in its basin that formed in the past, or to a new pattern that is created by chaotic processes which we experience as intuition. The set of basins forms an attractor landscape, and each new basin jostles the others as it forms. The second way is by reciprocal relations with all the other sensory cortices, mainly through the entorhinal cortex. Corollary discharges by preafferent pathways can bias the attractor landscapes of the cortices, and this bias can enhance or occlude certain basins of attraction to conform to the goals emerging through the limbic system. How this occurs at the cellular level is grist for the reductionist mill, but the fact that it does occur is established by measurement and analysis of the local AM patterns that form during intention and its derivative through preafference, attention.

The receptors continually bombard the sensory cortices, and they bombard each other by pulse activity, irrespective of intention. Each module of the brain is subject to destabilization at any time owing to the impact of these pulses on its intrinsic dynamics. There must be some form of global coordination to explain the unity of intentional action and the perseverance of goal-directed states in the face of distractions and unexpected obstacles. My view is that the interactions of the neural populations create the global AM pattern of shared activity in each hemisphere. The populations are not locked together in synchronous discharge, because they preserve a high degree of autonomy. Synchrony seldom occurs among the individual neurons in the local populations, either. The entire communities of modules in the two hemispheres, cooperating through the brainstem, the corpus callosum and other interhemispheric commissures, express a single, global, dynamic framework. The micro–macro relation that binds single neurons in populations, then, is a precursor for the organization of the limbic and sensory systems into global brain states.

Because the global AM patterns consist of the widespread coordination of axonal pulses and dendritic waves, they are difficult to detect except by their impact on behaviours. At the moment, all we have are glimpses of the global brain activity. This sort of problem is familiar in many fields. For example, a tsunami is a giant tidal wave that can have catastrophic effects on coastal areas, but it is virtually undetectable in the open ocean owing to its great breadth and low height. In the field of economics, macroeconomic trends are experienced by individuals as affluence or unemployment, but they become clear only after economists have collected and analysed statistics showing that they are pervading the population. An entire culture can be collapsing into revolution, yet many of its people can remain blithely unaware that anything is wrong. Only the most astute political leaders can detect the emergence of new opportunities and the means to exploit them.

But once we have described and explained the global AM patterns detected by recordings of electric and magnetic fields of potential in and over the cerebral hemispheres, we still have to explain their relation to awareness. It seems to me that the global AM patterns we detect are the biological basis for awareness.

Each of the interactive populations of the brain is continually creating new local patterns of chaotic activity. Each population widely disseminates its activity and contributes to the trajectory of the global state. The constraint exercised by each module of the brain, acting on others by participating in the global AM pattern, diminishes the freedom of all of them, so the likelihood that any one of them will destabilize and impose its activity onto other modules is reduced. In particular, it is less likely that any one or a subset of modules can capture the motor systems and shape behaviours with minor contributions from other parts. The crucial role played by awareness, according to this hypothesis, is to prevent precipitous action not by inhibition, but by quenching local chaotic fluctuations through sustained interaction that acts as a global constraint for damping, as described by Prigogine. Chaotic fluctuations lead to order, but only those fluctuations that are directed towards an intended basin. Others are continually folded back into the noise, if the order parameter is strong enough to do that.

Only a small fraction of the total variance of the activity in each of the modules is incorporated into the global pattern, but those small parts are crucial. Just as an individual neuron is subject to continual bombardment at its synapses yet can only report out a pulse intermittently on its sole axon, and just as the population is built from the seemingly random activity of millions of neurons yet can form only one attractor pattern at a time, so the whole hemisphere, in achieving unity from its myriad shifting parts, can sustain only one global AM pattern at a time. And just as neurons retain their autonomy, so the local modules retain theirs. Their activities boil along under the gentle constraint of the whole, constituting what many people refer to as unconscious processing, and what James called the penumbra of the spotlight of consciousness. But consciousness is not a spotlight, because that would require a focused beam, whereas global AM patterns are non-local. Moreover, a spotlight requires some other mechanism to aim it, whereas the global AM pattern is self organizing. A closer mechanical metaphor, if any were needed, would be a thermostat that samples and regulates temperature.

Awareness, then, is a distributed event that integrates the component subsystems and minimizes the likelihood of renegade state transitions in them. Consciousness is the process that makes a sequence of global states of awareness. It is a state variable that constrains the chaotic activities of the parts by quenching local fluctuations. It is an order parameter and an operator that comes into play in the action–perception cycle as an action is being concluded, and as the learning phase of perception begins. This is the part of the intentional arc in which the consequences of a just-completed action are being organized and integrated into meaning, and a new action is being developed but is not yet being executed. This is how consciousness facilitates the enrichment of meaning. It holds back premature action and, by giving time for maturation and closure, it increases the likelihood of the expression in considered behaviour of the long-term promise of an intentional being.

This reminds me of something James wrote in 1879, when he was wrestling with the implications of Darwinian natural selection for brain function. In an article entitled 'Are we automata?', he asked whether consciousness might have a functional role that would endow its possessor with a competitive edge. The opposing view was that consciousness is an epiphenomenon by which we might know God and feel pleasure or pain, but without affecting the activities of the neurons producing it. James concluded that consciousness is 'an organ added for the sake of steering a nervous system grown too complex to regulate itself'. But it is not an organ in the sense of some part of a brain, such as the frontal lobe, the amygdala, or the midbrain reticular formation, or a nucleus in the brainstem. It is a higher level of self organization.

This insight follows from having to wrestle with two kinds of brain structure. One is the anatomical architecture of brains, which continues to surprise us as we learn more about how brains work. The other is the dynamic architecture of brain state space. We know far less about that than chemists know about the dynamics of biochemistry, and that physicists know about the pathways of particle formation. I have postulated only three

levels in a hierarchy, but there are good reasons to add more
levels, both below the neuron in the chemistry of synaptic membranes and the readout of the genome during learning, and above
the global state of the hemispheres to include self awareness
and the environment, especially the social encounters by which
individual brains assimilate meaning.

This view of consciousness as a dynamic operator offers some
insight into the issue of emotion versus reason. We can relate
the degree of emotion to the intensities of chaotic fluctuations
in the populations of the forebrain, which are regulated by the
neuromodulators secreted by brainstem nuclei under limbic
control. We can regard reason as expressing a high degree of
assimilation to the world, which is meaning based in extensive
knowledge that endows a rational mind with remarkable power.
Consciousness does not form the trajectory of reason. It provides
the global linkage for smoothing chaotic fluctuations through
interactions. By these criteria, an action can be intensely emotional and yet strictly constrained. Actions that we interpret as
thoughtless, ill-conceived, rash, incontinent, inattentive or even
unconscious, we can now describe in dynamics as being shaped
by the escape of local fluctuations from the global order parameter, prematurely in respect to unity, maximum grip, and
long-term growth towards wholeness of intentionality. Actions
that we describe as visionary and constructive are well constrained. Emotion and reason can rise and fall together or be
disparate. Incontinence is one form of disparity from a deficit of
constraint; apathy is another from a deficit of chaotic activity.

This analysis in terms of neurodynamics can help to explain
why the notion of free will remains elusive. A voluntary action
is clearly intentional, but it must proceed with awareness. Yet
when a person has chosen an action, he or she may not be the
first to become aware of the choice. Instead, observers of the
action may be the first to become aware of it and attribute agency
to the actor. Both the observers and the actor may understand the
self-organizing dynamics of brains as the source of intentional
actions, but, even if they do not grasp this, they attribute the
action correctly to the actor, although in all modesty the actor

may demur, and rightfully so, that the observed action may not have been what he or she had consciously intended.

The anomaly appears when brains are understood to be a material system subject to the laws of physics. Donald Davidson, a philosopher, questions:

Why on earth should a cause turn an action into a mere happening and a person into a helpless victim? Is it because we tend to assume, at least in the arena of action, that a cause demands a causer, agency and agent? So we press the question: if my action is caused, what caused it? If I did, then there is the absurdity of an infinite regress: if I did not, I am a victim. But of course the alternatives are not exhaustive. Some causes have no agents. Among these agentless causes are the states and changes of state in persons which, because they are reasons as well as causes, constitute certain events as free and intentional actions.

He answers his question by adopting a position he calls 'anomalous monism', for which he has two premises. First, all physical systems, including the brain, are subject to the deterministic, causal laws of physics. Second, meaning is an open system, because it is so obviously shared in societies. Davidson concludes that the capacity to make choices and implement meaning is undeniable to humans but is anomalous.

In my view, both his premises have been undermined by new developments in physics and neurodynamics. First, what he thinks of is classical physics within the framework of linear causality: closed physical systems that go to equilibrium at point attractors. Dead brains do that, but living brains are open systems that feed on energy and freely dispose waste and heat. As such, they are capable of self-organizing chaotic dynamics that leads to unpredictable and complex new behaviours. Second, meaning is constructed within each brain as a closed system because of solipsistic isolation. Meaning only appears to be an open system because of the mechanisms of social assimilation, which we will look at in Chapter 7.

The denial of free will, then, comes from viewing a brain as being embedded in a linear causal chain. Because linear causality is the product of the intentional mechanism by which brains construct knowledge, and because it is misplaced when assigned to complex material systems, the apposition of free will against determinism creates a pseudo-problem. No intentional action is free of its historical context, nor is it entirely constrained by genetic and environmental determinants. The nature–nurture deterministic dyad – a sort of Aristotelian law of the excluded middle – fails to take into account the capacity for intentional beings to construct and pursue their individual goals within the contexts of their societies. Even when their genetic endowments are indistinguishable, as among identical twins, individuals choose unique directions in which to develop their realizable potentials. If the choices are attributed to random noise, then that is a confession of assigning no knowable cause. In other words, free will and universal determinism are irreconcilable boxes to which linear causality leads, and the only ways out of them are to deny freedom by assuming randomness, or to deny cause except as an action in a social context by an intentional being.

In summary, each of us is a source of meaning, a wellspring for the flow of fresh constructions within our brains and bodies, sheltered by the privacy of isolation. Our constructions are by the exuberant growth of patterns of neural activity from the chaotic dynamics of populations containing myriads of neurons. Our intentional actions continually flow into the world, changing the world and the relations of our bodies to it. This dynamic system is the self in each of us. It is the agency in charge, not our awareness, which is constantly trying to catch up with what we do. We perceive the world from inside our boundaries as we engage it and then change ourselves by assimilation. Our actions are perceived by ourselves and others as the pursuit of individual goals, and as the expression of our meanings by gestures, signs, words and numbers; that is, by representations.

But how does the self perceive itself? Is there any more to it than the recollections of experiences that are bound together in the unity of intentionality? Self awareness implies yet another level of organization above that of consciousness, a level that exists only in humans and to a very limited extent in some of our closest relatives, the great apes. The difference in organization of brain state space must in some way be related to the difference in organization of the anatomical brain between humans and more distant animals. The best place to start looking is in differences in the relations between the limbic system and the vast areas of the frontal and temporal lobes that were added to human brains in the past half a million years of evolution.

According to Larry Squire and others, the medial temporal lobes, which enclose the hippocampus and entorhinal cortex, are necessary in humans for the formation of explicit memories that we can consciously recall. This kind of learning is distinct from classical conditioning of behaviour, by which we can learn without being aware of the process and the outcome or being able to recall them. We call the process subliminal conditioning, and the memories that it forms are implicit. The limbic system, by virtue of its multimodal convergence and divergence, its control of brainstem nuclei, and its privileged access to the space–time field of the brain, appears to have evolved as the main conduit and locus of integration of neural activities into awareness. It seems to facilitate access to basins of the global attractor that mediate the unity of momentary experience. But consciousness and self consciousness do not reside there, nor in the frontal lobes, nor yet in any other delimited parts of the brain.

Chapter 7

Knowledge and meaning in societies

How does public knowledge differ from private meaning? On the one hand, my experimental work leads me to think that all humans and other animals are isolated within themselves by the mechanisms of biological intelligence. This is an essential condition for intentional existence, and the reason is clear. The material world we cohabit is infinitely rich in details, far beyond the capacity of even the most powerful mind to grasp except in small but sufficient fragments. We shape ourselves in coming to terms with those portions, not by imbibing them, but by assimilating to them through hypothesis testing. All that we can know and carry as meaning is the sum of the hypotheses and the results of the tests. But on the other hand, humans are first and foremost social animals. The most obvious fact of biological evolution in the past half million years is that the forms and dynamics of our brains and bodies have grown and adapted through social communication and interaction. This effort has been a magnificent response to the challenge posed by solipsistic isolation. No nuclear family can amount to more than a pride of lions or a pod of whales without the biological machinery that has emerged and adapted for the representation of meanings in social contexts. The adaptation includes the face, larynx, tongue and hyoid bones, the hands and the brain systems necessary for making and reading the required gestures, grimaces and utterances, and the glorious symbols and images we find inscribed on the walls of caves and rock shelters on every continent, which are the precursors of writing and computer graphics.

Private meaning that is represented to others becomes public knowledge when it has been perceived and assimilated by others as a basis for communal action. It is the dialectical tension between our solipsistic isolation and the requirement for us to surmount it that informs both neurobiology and sociobiology. Brains do not make sense when they are viewed in the context of linear causality as computational systems for representation, communication and command. Models of social systems based on information processing by genes, pheromones, stratified collectives, and chemomechanical energy transfers are reasonable for ants and termites, up to a point, but for humans they are absurd. Many economists and political theorists are aware of the need for better models of human behaviour than those provided by sociobiologists, but neurobiologists have not been helpful in efforts to meet that need in the past half-century. I think we can do better, at the very least to remove the dead hand of socio-genetic determinism. If voluntary choice is respectable in neurobiology, why not in sociobiology?

Individual minds, with their isolated meanings, assimilate to each other and create transcendent social entities that enhance and empower the individuals. Some people like to call these entities 'group minds'. There is some justification for this in terms of shared knowledge and joint action, but they cannot have group awareness because there is no interconnecting material substrate, and I will not accept a mechanism based on extra-sensory perception, quantum nonlocality or any other media for brain-to-brain communication between people. These cannot possibly work because of the unidirectional operation of intentionality. The term 'society' suffices, whether it refers to a family, a tribe, an urban gang, a tong, a church, a scientific assembly, a political party, a corporation or an economic entity, all of which are invariably organized around some form of representation such as a crest, a shield, a sign, a totem, an emblem, a flag, an icon, a logo, or a letterhead.

The model I propose for social self organization is an extension of the micro–macro interactions we saw between neurons and populations, and between populations and global AM patterns. In each level, the individual retains autonomy but accepts constraint in respect to the embedding surround. Failure of individual autonomy leads to apathy and stagnation. Failure of constraint leads to anarchy and disintegration. The archetypal experience is with the committee, struggling for consensus in the face of boredom, obstinacy and conflicting purposes, dissolving pent-up resentments with banter and laughter. We shall have a look at some of the neurobiological aspects of these micro–macro interactions between individuals and societies, in the hope that neurobiologists may contribute something useful after all to dialogues with the social sciences.

In the preceding chapters, we examined the biological foundation of meaning as an expression of the particular situation of an individual. Meaning emerges in sequences of global AM patterns of oscillatory neural activity coordinating the neuropil of an entire cerebral hemisphere. The amplitude of the oscillations is high in local patches and low in others, as viewed through brain imaging, in which, as with all patterns, both the highs and lows are necessary. Each pattern is a construction of the brain, with onset and termination by global state transitions. The contributions to the pattern are both local and large scale. Local details are provided by synapses that have been modified by previous learning and now shape local bursts as they emerge in patches of the forebrain, including the primary sensory cortices, the limbic system, and the brainstem nuclei. The interactions of these patches with each other and with the brainstem create a global state, which organizes and constrains local activity in a process of circular causality. At any given time, this state – which is constantly in flux as individuals grow and learn – is the meaning in a person.

Humans, as social beings, have assimilated meanings from one another. Each member of a society constantly learns through intentional action and learning, so that his or her behaviours become increasingly predictable, intelligible and mutually supportive for others. We adopt these forms of meaning through educational, religious and military institutions, in which many people participate and which are tools for activity in concert. The distinction we will make in this chapter – between private meaning and public knowledge – concerns the source of meanings, not what meanings contain. Both private meanings and the assimilated meanings that are derived through knowledge exist as patterns in brains and, in the biological sense, they are exactly the same, although each is a small fraction of the other. But in order to integrate biological insights so we can understand the social nature of human beings, we need to distinguish between private meaning, which comes by individual action into the environment, and meaning learned through interaction with others. Although there are no clear boundaries separating private and assimilated meaning within individuals, the distinction is useful for analysing social phenomena.

How can private meaning be assimilated to the meanings in others when it incorporates the entirety of a person's past experience? Each brain forms a world unto itself by continually constructing actions through its body into the world. Given the richness and complexity of this fabric of past growth and the unique potential of each individual, it makes no sense to infuse or inject meaning from one brain to another. The boundary enclosing the unity of each organism cannot be penetrated without disrupting the organism, causing it to heal itself by learning. But assimilation is normal: when it fails, individuals may become rigid and demonstrate repetitious behaviours in abnormal states, which form a class of diseases known as dynamic psychiatric diseases, including psychomotor epilepsy, hallucinations, Tourette's syndrome, obsessive–compulsive disorder, and Parkinson's disease. We can also include in this group the abrupt and unpredictable switching between multiple personalities, as a dissociation of global attractor landscapes into several fragments. We normally create within ourselves assimilated states with uninterrupted accumulations of episodic memories of others by observing and interpreting their actions, which we experience as empathy. We confirm our similarity by shared gestures and words of joy, condolence, threat and invitations to cooperate. Our isolation provides the gift of privacy, but also the curse of loneliness. Most of us have an intense desire to understand others and to be understood. We respond by making ourselves similar to each other; this is assimilation.

Two extreme forms of the relation between individuals and their society have been envisaged by Émile Durkheim and other cultural anthropologists. At one pole are societies in which members are deeply integrated, such that thoughts and behaviours between them conform exceedingly closely, and even the existence of private consciousness may be inconceivable to the participants. At the other extreme are societies in which individuals are autonomous to the point of anarchy. Durkheim's 'anomie' refers to those temporary periods between the breakdown of one social order and the organization of its replacement, when individuals are not tightly constrained by social norms: they lack a great deal of assimilated meaning. (Such interludes have the same characteristics as chaotic state transitions in brains, notably premonitory fluctuations building from disorder into order, which Tani believes are the only times in which the self exists.) But the societies can last for a long time because there is a balance between total conformity and total anarchy. Stability at the cost of rigidity is attained with a high proportion of assimilated meaning, whereas flexibility at the cost of unpredictability and chaos comes from a high proportion of private meaning. Given the varieties of predictable and unpredictable rates of environmental change in the world, it would be futile to try to define any perfect balance between the glacial hyperstability of social evolution under a corporate mentality and the catastrophic instability of unfettered individualism.

Every intentional act is an expression of the internal state of meaning in the brain and body. An act becomes a representation of the internal state when it is intentionally directed towards another person. There must be an intent to solicit the formation of a similar state of meaning in the other person, which might then be confirmed by a reciprocal intentional act. But there is no need for either party to be aware of this. The only requirement is a goal-directed state that is expressed in shared action if the communication is successful, whether the outcome is making love or war. This is shown in Figure 2 to represent an exchange between two humans, but it can be generalized to include communication between people and different species as well, because many animals make recognizable intentional gestures, such as courtship displays in mating. Social animals use facial expressions and body language to communicate their internal states and intended actions to others of their kind. In Charles Darwin's book *The Expression of Emotions in Man and Animals* (1878), he described the remarkable similarities across species in the techniques used to convey intentional states involving dominance and submission in the competition for food, mates and shelter.

As Darwin pointed out, these gestures are evolutionary adaptations to new uses of postural and autonomic support systems for actions needed to satisfy the basic needs of living and reproduction. One of the best sources is the repertoire for temperature regulation, which includes shivering, panting, blushing and the erection of hair for insulation by a fur coat, which gives hairless humans goose-bumps. But preparations are not always followed by actions. An animal can withhold or delay its intended action, leaving in place its emotional gesture as a signal to others of the continued possibility of attack or escape. The signal can be read by others through experiences with behaviours that are stored in chaotic attractor landscapes by neural mechanisms determined by genes and the laws of embryological development. When the global brain state settles into an appropriate basin in the landscape of the motor systems, the signalling behaviour governed by the attractor is stable enough to be received across generations and even species.

Like the components making up bodily motion and feeding, the structures of signalling behaviours are constrained by the genome. Learning and practice are required to perfect both the expression of gestures and their perception and correct interpretation. We observe this training every day in the play of children, kittens, puppies and other young mammals. Again, awareness of exchanges is not needed for communication to be effective, but learning is essential to control and read gestures.

We cannot know whether animals and children immersed in a world of play and practice in their imaginations are aware of what they are doing, but we know that, as adults, we can often give our best performances when we are not aware of our actions or ourselves, only of our goals. Good artists know how to keep their egos in check until the work is done.

Humans, of course, have advanced substantially beyond the use of gestures. We cut, mould and weave objects from all sorts of materials, paint walls with coloured pigments, and cut away at mountains to make representations. These images express admiration, fear, prediction, desire for a mate, sexual satisfaction, killing an animal, defeating an enemy, or finding a heaven beyond pain and suffering. The records on the walls of caves around the world show how images have evolved from stick figures and handprints into geometrical forms representing animals, people in ceremonies, rain, phases of the moon, crops and tools. The symbols became more complex as abstractions representing life, death, resurrection and the interchangeable spirits of animals and ancestors. To modern witnesses, such as archaeologists and palaeontologists, the artists' intent seems to have been to understand and communicate with unknown powers in order to placate and control them, but it is far too late for researchers to assimilate their meanings through cooperative action with the artists. Now we can only speculate about what the material representations meant to the tribal artists who made them, because they have no meaning, and they never did. In accordance with concepts from Thomas Aquinas, meanings exist only in minds, not in objects. Human artefacts are instruments that people use to instigate the creation of meaning in other people. They are neither vehicles that carry meaning nor reservoirs that store it for future generations. Objects can be used to store and transmit data, but information is not meaning. The evidence is that the geometric forms endure, but the meanings in the minds of modern archaeologists inevitably differ from the meanings in the minds of the prehistoric tribesmen who created the artefacts.

The further transition of representational skills to language, followed by the development of ideographic and alphabetic representations of spoken phonemes, syllables and words, is relatively trivial, in the same sense that the controlled release of nuclear energy is only a step beyond the subjugation of fire. Without being compelled to commit ourselves to expensive, dangerous and irremediable situations, our linguistic skills enable us to predict and play out scenarios of actions for practice to evaluate probable consequences. Linguists and neuro-scientists are dedicated to analysing the brain mechanisms responsible for making and understanding language, and rightly so, as these skills underlie the social organizations that make humans pre-eminent among animal species on Earth. But it is unlikely that these mechanisms can be understood without first clarifying the biological basis for intentionality. Followers of Noam Chomsky need look no further than the action–perception cycle in the brain for the 'deep structure' of the subject–verb–object relations in various languages, as it is the intentional arc of brain and body that languages emulate.

Reading the nuances of others' expressions allows us to see only the surface of the deep ocean of meaning that lies within each of us. Even after growing up with a sibling, or after living and working with another person for years, we base our cooperative action with them on trust, not on complete knowledge. Trust is the unquestioning acceptance of another person as being what he or she appears to be, rather like the belief that the person you go to sleep with at night will be the same when you both wake up. Because of trust, we can reasonably predict the behaviour of people we know well. We 'understand' them, in that the ways in which they act and express themselves closely match our expectations. Communication by representations is quite limited, considering what little impact images and words often have in rendering the complexity, stability and dynamic inertia of personalities we trust. This is simply an aspect of our solip-sistic isolation. Another aspect is that the nature of our learning processes makes us more and more isolated as we grow older, as our cumulative episodic meaning structures become more complex with time and experience. We grow apart because of our unique personal histories. The more we learn, the more specialized we become, and the less competent we are to understand one another. Even such strongly bonded pairs as parents and children may realize that they are strangers to one another as children leave home for work, college or their own mates.

The specializing and unquestioning adaptation that comes with cumulative learning is the norm in a stable environment, like that of a child in a successful family structure. The adaptation may fail when there is catastrophic change, such as a death in the family, which is inherently unpredictable and so cannot be met by Hebbian learning. Adaptation by learning also fails as a result of a major event that occurs in the normal life cycle of all mammals: the passage from being a child to becoming a competent adult and parent. This transition is so familiar and so deeply ingrained into human experience that it is difficult to step back and admire the process as a whole. It consists of a transfer of primary social attachment from parents to a new mate and one's own offspring. That transformation means that old habits, values, skills and beliefs must be given up to make way for new ones. In other words, there is a large-scale conversion of the intentional structure of meaning in the passage from child to adult.

Conventional processes of learning cannot account for this conversion, because such a radical change requires something other than just the growth of a new meaning structure on top of the old one. It seems to me that a unique process is necessary to dissolve the existing meaning structure and replace it with a new one that meets the requirements for social bonding in mammalian reproduction. I call this process 'unlearning' to distinguish it from forgetting or loss by fatigue, habituation, disuse or overlay by new connections. A good 'forgettory' is better than a good memory, because psychiatrists know that more people live in mental anguish because they cannot forget than because they cannot remember, but the process of unlearning is closer to forgiving than forgetting. Indeed, the most benign pathology of old age is presbyphrenia, defined in *Webster's* 3rd edition as 'a form of senile dementia occurring chiefly among women and characterized by loss of memory often to the point of disorientation with preservation of mobility, loquacity, good spirits, and considerable mental alertness'.

The process of unlearning first came under scientific scrutiny in the laboratory of Ivan Pavlov, who discovered techniques for drastically altering behaviour. Pavlov and his colleagues subjected their laboratory dogs to severe stress, including vigorous exercise, prolonged and excessive sensory stimulation, lack of sleep, isolation from normal social contacts, and strong emotional states of rage or fear. As a result of this overload, the animals reached a point at which they failed to respond at all and finally collapsed. Pavlov called this state 'transmarginal inhibition', in accordance with their theory of brain function based on grades of inhibition. Immediately after recovery from this collapse, the dogs were found to have lost all of their prior learning and had to be trained again. Because all of their former behavioural patterns were lost, they could be trained to perform in new ways without interference from old learning.

In his book *Battle for the Mind* (1958), the psychiatrist William Sargant described how the same techniques have been used by social authorities and institutions in many cultures over many centuries to bring about political and religious conversions. They have been known to tyrants and have been used for enslavement of subjects for thousands of years. Pavlov's work had merely given the procedures some physiological rationale. But the explication also did a disservice, because the techniques came to be labelled as 'brainwashing', which is widely seen as a vicious and oppressive method of compelling people to adopt behaviours and attitudes they would otherwise find repugnant. This is ironic, because what is lost in this condemnation is the recognition that these techniques, in less extreme and more invitational form, are not only widespread in modern societies, but are essential for the formation of cohesive social groups based on deep trust. They have been used in military camps, college fraternities and sororities (as 'hazing'), street gangs, sports teams, training programmes in large corporations to induce team spirit, and the arduous demands placed on students training for careers in law, medicine and the sciences. Life-long bonds, of the kind outsiders encounter as 'old-boy networks' and sisterhoods, are formed between those who have such deep emotional experiences with their peers.

Trust induced by unlearning can blanket vast gaps between small areas of assimilated meaning in the minds of believers. Young adults who have been cut adrift from their parents and siblings seek affiliations, not just for physical protection, but to find purpose, meaning and identity in their lives through shared actions. Recognizing this search helps us to understand the attraction of religious cults and urban street gangs, which flourish in defiance of the attempts by conventional social authorities to suppress or disperse them.

Pavlov's transmarginal inhibition demonstrates that extraordinary ordeals endured by individuals can selectively break down the stability of intentional architecture so that general knowledge, personal history, and language and motor skills, although briefly lost in the trance state, are soon regained, but social attitudes, values and goals are dissolved. This opens the way for the growth of new intentional structure, as long as social guidance and support are provided by the brainwashers. An ordeal may be based either on externally imposed stress or on developmental changes within the brain and body, of which puberty is the most important example. Virtually all human societies have rites of passage to help transform their young into full adult members of their groups. Tribal rituals of the kinds described by anthropologists are very similar to activities that have been used for centuries in social and religious conversions. They rely heavily on communal activities of dancing, chanting, clapping and swaying together for hours, or even days and nights. Overwhelmed by exhaustion and sensory overload, a participant eventually collapses into a state of transmarginal inhibition. The dancer is then carefully nurtured into recovery, sometimes after being carried to a graveyard and symbolically 'brought back to life' in a ritual re-enactment of death and rebirth. Social support and constraining joint actions are then crucial for re-education in new values.

Rhythmic drumming and music are almost universal in these

rites. People often use them to lose self awareness and induce
an altered state of consciousness, which they experience as transport and observers see as a trance. For millennia, wine, tobacco,
mushrooms, jimson weed and cacti have been used to induce
such trances. Young people in modern societies use an amphetamine derivative, Ecstasy, in conjunction with techno music
and rave dancing in their search for feelings of community and
bonding. The role of music is particularly important, as the
strong sense of knowing when the next beat will come, and of
impending closure in the resolution of a diminished seventh,
grabs and holds us as no other language can. Acting together is
the basis for trusting each other, and there are few stronger and
more intimate form of joint action than dancing to a common
beat. The variety and ubiquity of neuromodulators suggests that
unlearning, which is a prelude to learning new assimilated meanings through cooperative action, is brought about by the release
of one or more neuromodulators in the brain. It seems to me
that the action of such chemicals can loosen the synaptic fabric
of the neuropil and open the way to global change. An example
of this is falling in love and remembering the song that was
playing.

A clue to the identity of these neuromodulators comes from
recent studies of the changes in mammalian brains that accompany reproductive behaviours. An important neurochemical that
has been implicated by behavioural neuropharmacologists such
as Thomas Insel in the process of synaptic change is oxytocin.
This neuromodulator has been known for many years, because
the brain releases it into the blood to induce labour in pregnant
women by stimulating the uterus and to induce lactation by
stimulating the mammary glands. But scientists have recently
discovered that oxytocin directly affects the forebrain, where it
is released during orgasm in sexual intercourse in both male
and female humans and other animals. Insel and his colleagues
showed that oxytocin is essential for pair-bonding in one of two
species of voles after mating. This species is characterized by
peaceful coexistence and monogamous pair-bonds, and the
brains in these animals are dominated by oxytocin. The other

species, in which vasopressin is dominant, rather than oxytocin, is characterized by promiscuity and aggressiveness. Studies of maternal behaviour in voles and other species show that oxytocin is released only briefly, and that it sets the stage for the formation of new behaviours, rather than being secreted steadily to maintain existing behaviours, which is the case for most other hormones, such as thyroid and estrogen.

In sheep, oxytocin is released in the olfactory bulb when a mother delivers her young, but if its action is blocked, the mother fails to bond with them. Bonding between mother and offspring in many animals is accomplished primarily by imprinting to body scents, but oxytocin is not released in the delivery of the first litter, only in the second and later litters. This implies that oxytocin is required to expunge an olfactory imprint from a previous litter to pave the way for the imprinting of a new one. In other words, there needs to be unlearning of old meaning before new meaning can form, without significant loss of the procedural motor skills and episodic memories of experience. The process of unlearning is a remarkable achievement of biological and cultural evolution of mammals.

The neural machinery enabling the process of unlearning probably comes from the genome of mammals, for whom reproduction requires prolonged care of dependent offspring. The mother and father must bond to them, as well as to one another. Pair-bonds form at birth, during lactation, and in sexual arousal and union. These processes are outstanding examples of intentionality at work, in the unity of action, perception, experience, learning and maturation of the brain and body, all directed through the individual choice of partners towards the realization of the full potential of the participants. Humans have the same neural machinery to support pair-bonding of adults with each other and with children. It seems to me that humans have discovered how to control unlearning through trance states, using techniques of behavioural modification for bonding far beyond the range of the nuclear family and the tribe. These practices have been elaborated through cultural evolution and are pervasive in modern societies, although their social significance goes largely unnoticed and their neurochemical bases are largely undocumented.

Socialization and acculturation are life-long processes, but are particularly intensive in the first days and years of life. To account for the unlearning, however small it may be, that necessarily occurs in our daily lives, I suggest that unlearning happens every night during sleep through the release of the requisite neuromodulators. Such an idea fits well with the observation that young people, who display very high rates of learning, unlearning and re-education, spend a high proportion of their time in REM sleep. The young, in particular, need to unlearn and learn constantly as they prepare to participate fully in the social world and accept the gift of cultural knowledge provided by the educational process. With the rare exceptions of so-called 'wild children', who have somehow survived infancy and grown to adolescence without social contact, every human is nurtured and shaped through years of repeated cycles of dissolution and rebirth. Unfortunately, we know little about the neurochemistry of these cycles, the brain dynamics by which they are induced and ended, and the way that recently learned material is selected for retention, integration or dismissal, under the direction of the emergent intentional experience of each individual.

Failures in the developmental process have radical effects. Autism is a syndrome in which individuals develop no comprehension of the feelings, needs or emotions of their families and acquire no friends. Although some may become 'savants', possessing amazing talents for very specific activities such as arithmetic or remembering trivia, they are forever locked out of the assimilated meanings shared by others. Autistic children illustrate the outcome that, left unbridled and unchecked, the process of Hebbian learning can create isolated towers of complex meaning, but that the meaning remains unvalued and insignificant for the societies in which these individuals must live. An opposite pattern, called Williams syndrome, is found in children who are excessively malleable and responsive to others. They are unable to sustain organized effort towards long-term goals, such as getting an education and building a family, and they tend to assimilate with those with whom they have most recently interacted.

In conclusion, each brain, and the mind that is its function, is a unity that is isolated within a solipsistic barrier. This is a barrier only in the sense of a horizon, which endlessly recedes as it is approached. It is a texture that does not accept darning patches from the meanings of others. You cannot directly experience the qualia and meanings that exist in another brain, nor can any outsider enter into your own private world. You have to learn to understand and unlearn to empathize. But, as John Donne wrote, 'No man is an Island, intire of itselfe: every man is a peece of the Continent, a part of the maine' (Devotions, XVII). Everyone who reaches maturity has experienced the intense crucible of endlessly repeated transformations during infancy, childhood and adolescence. Human intentionality is not optimally productive and effective until it has been acculturated through a long educational process, by which the capacity emerges for cooperative social action based on a high degree of shared perception and understanding, or knowledge. Brainwashing is an adult form of transformation, suitable for managing existential midlife crises in political and religious arenas. In these circumstances it usually fails, because individuals cannot adapt completely to new social norms. We all retain the capacity for unique perspectives and unexpected actions, even if they are not exercised. Our brains are the foundry of new meanings, which come into our awareness when they are already self organized, after which we may choose to publish them in representations such as books, poems or movies, as a means of sharing them with others as new knowledge. Or we may choose to revise, defer or remain silent out of respect, humility, trepidation or laziness, but these are reasons and excuses, not causal agents. The biological capacity to make choices, and suffer the consequences, is, as Thomas Jefferson put it, inalienable. We cannot surrender it, even when we want to.

Bibliography

Background reading

Abraham, F.D., Abraham, R.H., Shaw, C.D. & Garfinkel, A. (1990) *A Visual Introduction to Dynamical Systems Theory for Psychology* (Aerial, Santa Cruz, CA).

Bloom, F.E. & Lazerson, A. (1988) *Brain, Mind, and Behavior* (2nd edn), (Freeman, New York).

Damasio, A.R. (1994) *Descartes' Error: Emotion, Reason, and the Human Brain* (Putnam, New York).

Freeman, W.J. (1992) Tutorial in neurobiology: From single neurons to brain chaos. *International Journal of Bifurcation and Chaos* 2, 451–482.

Freeman, W.J. (1975) *Mass Action in the Nervous System* (Academic, New York).

Freeman, W.J. (1995) *Societies of Brains. A Study in the Neroscience of Love and Hate* (Lawrence Erlbaum, Mahwah, NJ).

Gloor, P. (1997) *The Temporal Lobe and the Limbic System* (Oxford University Press, New York).

Pert, C.B. (1997) *Molecules of Emotion: Why You Feel the Way you Feel* (Scribner, New York).

Sargant, W.W. (1957) *Battle for the Mind* (Greenwood, Westport, CT).

Thelen, E. & Smith, L.B. (1994) *A Dynamic Systems Approach to the Development of Cognition and Action* (MIT Press, Cambridge, MA).

References mentioned in the text

Abeles, M. (1991) *Corticonics: Neural Circuits of the Cerebral Cortex* (Cambridge University Press).

Aquinas, St Thomas (1272) Treatise on Man. In *Summa Theologica*. (Translated by Fathers of the English Dominican Province; revised by

Sullivan, D.J. Great Books, Vol. 19 (William Benton) (Encyclopedia Britannica, Chicago, 1952).

Baars, B.J. (1997) *In the Theater of Consciousness: The Workspace of the Mind* (Oxford University Press, New York).

Barrie, J.M., Freeman, W.J. & Lenhart, M. (1996) Modulation by discriminative training of spatial patterns of gamma EEG amplitude and phase in neocortex of rabbits. *Journal of Neurophysiology* 76, 520–539.

Basar, E. (1998) *Brain Function and Oscillations* (Springer, Berlin).

Bellugi, U., Lichtenberger, L., Mills, D., Balaburda, A. & Korenberg, J. R. (1999) Bridging cognition, the brain, and molecular genetics: Evidence from Williams syndrome. *Trends in Neurosciences* 5, 197–207.

Braitenberg, V. & Schüz, A. (1991) *Anatomy of the Cortex: Statistics and Geometry* (Springer, Berlin).

Bressler, S.L., Coppola, R. & Nakamura, R. (1993) Episodic multiregional cortical coherence at multiple frequencies during visual task performance. *Nature* 366, 153–156.

Calvin, W.H. (1996) *The Cerebral Code. Thinking a Thought in the Mosaics of the Mind* (MIT Press, Cambridge, MA).

Cannon, W. (1939) *The Wisdom of the Body* (Norton, New York).

Clancey, W.J. (1993) Situated action: A neuropsychological interpretation response to Vera and Simon. *Cognitive Science* 17, 87–116.

Clark, A. (1996) *Being There. Putting Brain, Body, and World Together Again* (MIT Press, Cambridge, MA).

Clark, R.E. & Squire, L.R. (1998) Classical conditioning and brain systems: The role of awareness. *Science* 280, 77–81.

Conel, J.L. (1939–1967) *The Postnatal Development of the Human Cerebral Cortex* (Harvard University Press, Cambridge, MA).

Darwin, C. (1872) *The Expression of Emotion in Man and Animals.* (Murray, London).

Davidson, D. (1980) Actions, reasons, and causes. In *Essays on Actions and Events* (Clarendon, Oxford).

Dewey, J. (1914) Psychological doctrine in philosophical teaching. *Journal of Philosophy* 11, 505–512.

Diamond, M.C. & Hopson, J. (1998) *Magic Trees of the Mind: How to Nurture Your Child's Intelligence, Creativity, and Healthy Emotions from Birth through Adolescence* (Dutton, New York).

Dumenko, V.N. (1970) Electroencephalographic investigation of cortical relationships in dogs during formation of a conditioned reflex stereotype. In Rusinov V.S. (editor) *Electrophysiology of the Central Nervous System* (ed. Rusinov, V.S.; translated by Haigh, B., translation editor, Doty, R.W.) 107–118. (Plenum, New York).

Freeman, W.J. (1979) Nonlinear gain mediating cortical stimulus-response relations. *Biological Cybernetics* **33**, 237–247.

Freeman, W.J. & Schneider, W. (1982) Changes in spatial patterns of rabbit olfactory EEG with conditioning to odors. *Psychophysiology* **19**, 44–56.

Gibson, J.J. (1979) *The Ecological Approach to Visual Perception* (Houghton Mifflin, Boston).

Goldstein, K. & Gelb, A. (1939) The Organism: A Holistic Approach to Biology Derived From Pathological Data in Man (American, New York).

Grossberg, S. (ed.) (1988) *Neural Networks and Natural Intelligence* (MIT Press, Cambridge, MA).

Haken, H. (1983) *Synergetics: An Introduction* (Springer, Berlin).

Hebb, D.O. (1949) *The Organization of Behavior* (Wiley, New York).

Hendriks-Jansen, H. (1996) *Catching Ourselves in the Act: Situated Activity, Interactive Emergence, Evolution and Human Thought* (MIT Press, Cambridge, MA).

Herrick, C.J. (1948) *The Brain of the Tiger Salamander* (University of Chicago Press).

Hume, D. (1739) *Treatise on Human Nature* (Noon, London).

Hunter, E. (1956) *Brainwashing. The Story of Men Who Defied It* (Farrar, Straus, New York).

Insel, T.R. (1992) Oxytocin: A neuropeptide for affiliation. Evidence from behavioral, receptor autoradiographic, and comparative studies. *Psychoneuroendocrinology* **17**, 3–35.

James, W. (1879) Are we automata? *Mind* **4**, 1–21.

Jacobs, L.F. (1994) Natural space-use patterns and hippocampal size in kangaroo rats. *Brain, Behavior and Evolution* **44**, 125–132.

Kay, L.M. & Freeman, W.J. (1998) Bidirectional processing in the olfactory-limbic axis during olfactory behavior. *Behavioral Neuroscience* **112**, 541–553.

Koffka, K. (1935) *Principles of Gestalt Psychology* (Harcourt Brace, New York).

Köhler, W. (1940) *Dynamics in Psychology* (Grove, New York).

Klüver, H. & Bucy, P. (1939) Preliminary analysis of functions of the temporal lobe in monkeys. *Archives of Neurology and Psychiatry* **42**, 979–1000.

Lehmann, D., Ozaki, H. & Pal, I. (1987) EEG alpha map series: brain micro-states by space-oriented adaptive segmentation. *Electroencephalography and Clinical Neurophysiology* **67**, 271–288.

Lesse, H. (1957) Amygdaloid electrical activity during a conditioned response. *Proceedings of the 4th International Congress of EEG and Clinical Neurophysiology, Brussels*, 99–100.

Libet, B. (1994) *Neurophysiology of Consciousness: Selected Papers and New Essays* (Birkhauser, Boston, MA).

Llinás, R. & Ribary, U. (1993) Coherent 40 Hz oscillations characterize dream state in humans. *Proceedings of the National Academy of Sciences (USA)* **90**, 2078–2081.

Maclean, P.D. (1969) *The Triune Brain* (Plenum, New York).

Magoun, H.W. (1962) *The Waking Brain* (2nd edn) (Thomas, Springfield, IL).

Mark, V.H. & Ervin, F.R. (1970) *Violence and the Brain* (Harper and Row, New York).

Mark, V.H., Ervin, F.R. & Sweet, W.H. (1972) Deep temporal lobe stimulation in man. In *The Neurobiology of the Amygdala* (ed. Eleftherion, B.E.) 485–507 (Plenum, New York).

Merleau-Ponty, M. (1945/1962) *Phenomenology of Perception* (translated by Smith, C.) (Humanities, New York).

Merleau-Ponty, M. (1942/1963) *The Structure of Behavior* (translated by Fischer, A.L.) (Beacon, Boston, MA).

Miltner, W. H. R., Barun, C., Arnold, M., Witte, H. & Taub, E. (1999) Coherence of gamma-band EEG activity as a basis for associative learning. *Nature* **397**, 434–436.

Müller, M.M. *et al.* (1996) Visually induced gamma band responses in human EEG – A link to animal studies. *Experimental Brain Research* **112**, 96–112.

Nicolelis, M.A.L. *et al.* (1988) Simultaneous encoding of tactile information by three primate cortical areas. *Nature Neuroscience* **1**, 621–630.

Narabayashi, H. (1972) Stereotaxic amygdaloidotomy. In *The Neurobiology of the Amygdala* (ed. Eleftherion, B.E.) 459–483. (Plenum, New York).

Nicolelis, M. A. L. *et al.* (1988) Simultaneous encoding of tactile information by three primate cortical areas. *Nature Neuroscience* **1**, 621–630.

Nunez, P.L. (1995) *Neocortical Dynamics and Human EEG Rhythms* (Oxford University Press, New York).

O'Keefe, J. & Nadel, L. (1978) *The Hippocampus as a Cognitive Map* (Clarendon, Oxford).

Panksepp, J. (1998) *Affective Neuroscience: The Foundations of Human and Animal Emotions* (Oxford University Press).

Pedersen, C.A., Caldwell, J.D., Jirikowski, G.F. & Insel, T.R. (1992) Oxytocin in maternal, sexual, and social behaviors. *Annals of the New York Academy of Sciences* **652**, xi.

Penrose, R. (1994) *Shadows of the Mind* (Oxford University Press).

Piaget, J. (1930) *The Child's Conception of Physical Causality* (Harcourt Brace, New York).

Pribram, K. (1971) *Languages of the Brain: Experimental Paradoxes and Principles in Neuropsychology* (Prentice-Hall, Englewood Cliffs, NJ).

Prigogine, I. (1980) *From Being to Becoming: Time and Complexity in the Physical Sciences* (Freeman, San Francisco).

Reynolds, S. (1998) *Generation Ecstasy. Into the World of Techno and Rave Culture* (Little, Brown, New York).

Rodriguez, E. *et al.* (1999) Perception's shadow: Long-distance synchronization of human brain activity. *Nature* **397**, 430–433.

Roland, P.E. (1993) *Brain Activation* (Wiley-Liss, New York).

Sheer, D.E. (1989) Sensory and cognitive 40-Hz event-related potentials: Behavioral correlates, brain function, and clinical application. In *Brain Dynamics* (eds Basar, E. & Bullock, T.H.) 339–374. (Springer, Berlin).

Singer, W. & Gray, C. M. (1995) Visual feature integration and the temporal correlation hypothesis. *Annual Review of Neuroscience* **18**, 555–586.

Smart, A. *et al.* Spatio-temporal analysis of multi-electrode cortical EEG of awake rabbit. *Society for Neuroscience Abstracts* **189**, 13.

Smart, A. *et al.* (1997) Spatio-temporal analysis of multi-electrode cortical EEG of awake rabbit. Abstract, Society for Neuroscience, 189.13.

Tallon-Baudry, C., Bertrand, O., Delpuech, C. & Pernier, J. (1996) Stimulus-specificity of phase-locked and non phase-locked 40-Hz visual responses in human. *Journal of Neuroscience* **16**, 4240–4249.

Tallon-Baudry, C., Bertrand, O., Peronnet, F. & Pernier, J. (1998) Induced gamma-band activity during the delay of a visual short-term memory task in humans. *Journal of Neuroscience* **18**, 4244–4254.

Tani, J. (1998) An interpretation of the 'self' from the dynamical systems perspective: A constructivist approach. *Journal of Consciousness Studies* **5**, 516–542.

Taylor, J.G. (1997) Neural networks for consciousness. *Neural Networks* **10**, 1207–1225.

Tolman, E.C. (1948) Cognitive maps in rats and men. *Psychological Review* **55**, 189–208.

Tsuda, I. (1991) Chaotic itinerancy as a dynamical basis of hermeneutics in brain and mind. *World Futures* **32**, 167–184.

Watts, D.J. & Strogatz, S.H. (1998) Collective dynamics of 'small world' networks. *Nature* **394**, 440–442.

Index

Note: page references *in italic* refer to diagrams.

maps of the mind